# Quick Review of
# NEET PG 2022

AF825611

**Kamal KV** MBBS, MS (Orthopedics)
Ex-Senior Resident: Safdarjung, ESI – Okhla, Fortis – Noida
Ponseti and Ilizarov Techniques Fellow (Akola)
Madhya Pradesh – Indian Orthopedic Association
Hand Surgery Fellow (Pune), Maharashtra, India

***Foreign (Academic) Trips (Countries and Cities)***

Georgia (Tbilisi, Batumi)
Russia (Nalchik, Cheboksary, Stavropol, Kazan)
Kyrgyzstan (Jalalabad, Osh)
Nepal (Bharatpur, Bhairahawa, Dharan)
Ukraine (Vinnytsia, Kiev)
China (Ningbo, Nanchang, Nanning, Dali, Fuzhou, Guangzhou)
Belarus (Minsk)



**Peepee Publishers and Distributors (P) Ltd.**®

Quick Review of NEET PG 2022

*Published by*
**Pawaninder P. Vij and Anupam Vij**

Peepee Publishers and Distributors (P) Ltd.
***Head Office:*** 160, Shakti Vihar, Pitam Pura, Delhi-110 034 (India)

***Correspondence Address:***

**7/31, First Floor, Ansari Road, Daryaganj**
**New Delhi-110 002 (India)**

Ph: 41512412, 23246245, 9811156083

*e-mail:* peepee160@yahoo.co.in

*e-mail:* peepee160@gmail.com

**www.peepeepub.com**

**join us on facebook.com/pp.publishers**



**First Edition: 2022**

**ISBN:** 978-81-9523-443-1

## Dedicated to

I would like to dedicate this title to all those who arranged or served me during my foreign (academic) trips. I have tried my best to compile all the names (Sorry, if I forgoet someone to mention).

| S. No. | Countries | College | Credit to |
|---|---|---|---|
| 1 | **Georgia** | *i. Tbilisi* | Dr Amit Verma, Dr Swapna Chauhan, Dr Anish Acharya, Amaresh Panda, Anij |
| | | *ii. Batumi* | -"- |
| 2 | **Russia** | *iii. Nalchik* | Dr Sudhakar Tiwari, Dr Sumant Pandey, Dr Nishant Atri, Dr Gaurav Soni, Dr Madhav Sharma, Dr Hariom Sharma, Dr Saurabh, Dr Manas Awasthi, Dr Jawwad Ghodi |
| | | *iv. Cheboksary* | Dr Jitendra Gurjar, Dr Aquib Akhtar, Dr Navneet, Dr Sachin Verma |
| | | *v. Stavropol* | Dr Najeerul Ameen, Dr Anupam Mishra, Dr Divyesh |
| | | *vi. Kazan* | Dr Atul Shrivastav |
| 3 | **Kyrgyzstan** | *vii. Jalalabad* | Dr Shoaib Shahid, Dr Deepak, Dr Kishan Bhandari, Dr Deewakar Jha, Dr SP Saha, Dr Firoz, Dr Shubhayu, Dr Tahul Sinha, Dr Vidya, Dr Umar |
| | | *viii. Osh* | Dr Bhupendra Magarde, Dr Aftab, Dr Jitendra Chaurasiya |
| 4 | **Nepal** | *ix. Bhairahawa* | Dr Pranjal Kashiv, Dr Rahul Yadav, Dr Satyam Ojha |
| | | *x. Bharatpur* | Dr Sanket Dewan, Dr Gautam Solanki, Dr Akshay Gajipara |
| | | *xi. Dharan* | Dr Sandeep Chauhan |
| 5 | **Ukraine** | *xii. Vinnytsia* | Dr Jashan Preet Singh, Dr Ashray Khanna, Dr Ayush |
| | | *xiii. Kiev* | -"- |

| | | | |
|---|---|---|---|
| 6 | **China** | *xiv. Ningbo* | Dr Nimshad, Dr Jamshid, Dr Srikant |
| | | *xv. Nanchang* | Dr Azlan, Dr Khalid, Dr Armaan Ansari, Dr Prashant Raghuwanshi, Dr Ravi Singh, Dr Vishal Borana |
| | | *xvi. Nanning* | Dr Jazeer, Dr Pranay |
| | | *xvii. Dali* | Dr Kashif Agaz, Dr Mubasheer, Dr Mujahid Tyagi |
| | | *xviii. Fuzhou* | Dr Chinthu MR, Dr Pooja |
| | | *xix. Guangzhou* | Dr Abhimanyu, Dr Russi Singh |
| 7 | **Belarus** | *xx. Minsk* | Dr Rama Sah, Dr Varun Upadhyay |

# PREFACE

It gives me immense pleasure in releasing this book within such a short span of time (within one month of the exam, which was conducted on 20.05.2022).

Most of the questions are on recall basis and the content available on the social media has been utilized to the maximum. Since these are recall basis, so the questions may differ in terms of statement or the options, but every effort has been done to highlight the core topic, asked in the question.

Images may not be the same as asked in the exam. Moreover, I have chosen images with some arrows/ marks, so that the same can be described in the explanation. The students must know the identifying features of a given image/ histological slide.

Explanations are kept short and focusses more on the fact that why a particular option is the answer. Descriptive explanation is avoided so as to keep the title handy and easy to read and revise.

For the ease of studying, explanations are kept just after the question so that students can correlate the answer with the question. This is followed by the answer and the reference.

The basic purpose of this title is to give an idea about the pattern of examination, which is problem-based and clinical-oriented nowadays. Moreover, this title tries to highlight the important topics related to the exam.

I have tried my level best but some errors might have crept in despite my best efforts.

Some of the questions, I felt, were controversial. Moreover, different textbooks have different opinions (especially in clinical subjects), that adds to confusion. I hope, that students will pardon me in that case and will enjoy going through my work😊.

As I always say, that students are the best judge of my work, so please shower me with your valuable suggestions at **+91 84 7000 4333**. I am just a call/message away.

Happy reading and all the best for your future.

**Date: 10 June 2022**

**drkamalkv**
*E-mail:* **drkamalkvgroup**@gmail.com
*Website:* www.**drkamalkvgroup**.co.in
*Facebook:* **drkamalkvgroup**
*WhatsApp:* 84 7000 4333

## ACKNOWLEDGEMENTS

All thanks to Almighty (for imparting me with this passion of writing books and teaching), to my parents (for imparting qualities of a good human being), my brothers and sister (for giving me some wonderful memories of childhood), my wife (for supporting me in all my endeavours), my daughters (for allowing me to use their share of time with my students) and my dear students (for accepting my all titles with equal enthusiasm and also, who made me academically strong, to an extent).

Special thanks to **Mr. Pawaninder Paul Vij** sir and **Mr. Anupam Vij** sir for accepting all my work, without any hesitancy or objection.

Thanks are due for everyone behind this project, from the publication house.



**drkamalkv**
*E-mail:* **drkamalkvgroup**@gmail.com
*Website:* www.**drkamalkvgroup**.co.in
*Facebook:* **drkamalkvgroup**
*WhatsApp:* 84 7000 4333

## A BIG THANKS

With the entry of COVID-19, a major shift has been made from Offline to Online teaching. I would like to thank all the teachers, who are working hard to deliver the content in an online mode. It takes a lot of effort to create an online content. So, I feel, it's our duty to thank each and everyone, who are making teaching so convenient. Today, we can access the study matter 24×7.

I am teaching all the subjects singly, to Foreign Medical Graduates. Many times, I am not in a position to refer textbooks or sometimes, I have to prepare classes in a short span of time. At that time, I too, refer the videos of my favourite teachers.

## Drkamalkv's Personalized Classes

*Salient features:*

- Online mode only.
- Batch of **3-5 students** only.
- Individualized attention on each student.
- I will be teaching all the subjects singly.
- Preparation strictly as per the current pattern.
- Specially designed for foreign medical graduates.
- 2 separate courses:
    - FMGE/MCI screening exam
    - NExT/NEET-PG
- Students would be selected on the basis of '**early come, early serve**' basis.
- Monthly payment plans.
- Enquiries can be made at: +91 84 7000 4333

# IDEAL WAY OF PREPARING FOR NEET PG

One of my seniors, who lives in the room next to my room in the hostel, was preparing for State PG exam way back in 1998. Since he was staying next to me so, I used to help in lot of things so that he can focus only on studies. Also, I was supposed to appear in the State PG exam after 2 years, so I was interested in knowing his strategy as well.

I noticed that he was reading standard textbooks only. I was surprised a bit, because most of his batchmates were reading one SALGUNAN book, which was based on previous year MCQs. I asked him "Why are you following a different route"? He said, since he had read those textbooks during his MBBS days, so he is finding it very easy to revise them. He will go through that MCQ bank in the last 1 month before exam.

One year later, he appeared in State PG exam and he was no where in the merit list. Many of his friend who studied only MCQ bank (with relevant theory, pertaining to the answers) managed to get into the merit, though towards the later half of the merit-list.

I felt very sorry for him and I said to him "Sir, your strategy didn't work. You couldn't qualify". He was speechless but he said, no problem, I will try once more. I am not having shortage of time.

For next attempt, he decided to follow the same plan; 11 months for detailed study from standard textbooks and last 1 month for the MCQ bank. I was surprised. I said, "Why are u following this plan again, when it hadn't worked for you, the previous year"? He told me that in previous attempt, he read many things in detail, but couldn't revise them nicely in the end. During the exam, he was knowing many things, but because of lack of revision, he couldn't answer them correctly. So, it was a kind of failure of a proper study schedule. That may be because, it was his first attempt and he was not knowing the things properly. Now, since he had the experience, he will manage the things in a better way.

I was little hopeless about him. And I predicted that he will fail again, but to everyone's surprise, he scored 1st rank in State PG exam in the next attempt😊.

*Few things are very obvious from this true story:*

- You can score a good rank in PG exam only if you have read textbooks during your MBBS days nicely. The same you can then revise during your PG exam preparation.
- Nowadays we have so many image-based questions in the exam. Textbooks give you access to plenty of images, with keywords to identify that image. If you have read the textbooks nicely and have studied the images properly, you will never err during the exam.
- Proper planning of studies is very important in the time period before the exam. Keep only that much stuff, which you can revise easily before the exam. For most of the students (including me), memory (related to studies) lasts for few months, so we need regular revision. Reading once and leaving it, won't work. So, decide properly, what you wish to read and keep on reading that much study matter, till the end.

*Some more points:*

- Nowadays, we have many problem/clinical scenario-based questions. This emphasizes the need of attending your clinical postings sincerely during your MBBS days. If you have attended your ward postings properly, you will learn about the essentials of clinical diagnosis, the investigations done and the treatment plan for a particular case. Patients are the best teachers.
- During examination, once you have marked an answer, never change it. Most of the time, you will replace a right answer with a wrong answer.
- Last but not the least, a very practical advice. Please have a proper 8 hours sleep before the exam. I have myself witnessed the need of that. If your brain is fresh and active, you can solve around 10 more questions correctly. Usually, for many MCQs, we can rule out two options. We are stuck in the remaining two. So, to get to the final answer, one had to think a lot and for that our brain should be in fully alert mode. That is only possible, if brain has given proper rest for at least 8 hours.

These are my words. One can devise his own strategy depending on his/ her capabilities. But the basic principle remains the same. Whatever you read, revise it at least twice after the main reading. In simpler words, read less but revise more.

And don't forget to solve previous years MCQ bank.

# VOCAL FOR LOCAL

This concept of VOCAL for LOCAL came out during COVID time, but I was following it from my MBBS days. For every subject, I used to read textbooks written by Indian authors.

There were two reasons for this. Firstly, that I was a son of a JCO (of Indian army) and my father's salary was less than 10,000 per month (in 1990s) so I couldn't afford costlier textbooks and secondly my aim was to clear proff exams only. So, I preferred textbooks by Indian authors, which were little cheaper and easy to revise before exams (as they were not bulky enough).

Like for Physiology, my seniors told me to read Ganong/ Guyton, but I read Chaudhuri, for Pathology, they advised me to study Robbins, but I studied Harsh Mohan, for Medicine, they were in favour of Harrison, but I had gone for Alagappan, PJ Mehta and so on.

Even today, I prefer reading books by Indian authors. I am teaching all the subjects to Foreign Medical Graduates singly, and I find these textbooks very easy to read.

Even for this title, I have tried to take reference from Indian textbooks. I was trying to figure out whether these Indian textbooks hold any relevance in terms of PG exam or not. To my surprise, I found proper explanation (pertaining to the answer) for nearly 95% of the MCQs.

I am not against the worldwide recognized textbooks, but what I am trying to say is that, if you are not able to read those, at least do read textbooks by Indian authors and read them thoroughly. For example, many students (including me) are not able to read whole Harrison for Medicine, but we can read at least Alagappan, PJ Mehta etc.

Also, please don't consider Indian author's textbooks, inferior to any Western author's textbooks. May be, being an Indian, I am advocating too much for Indian author's textbooks😊.

The final word is that studies are important. One can choose the title as per his/her capability.

The various Indian textbooks, which I have used as reference textbooks for answering MCQs are as follows:

**Anatomy:**

- Title 1: Inderbir Singh's Textbook of Anatomy, 6th edition, Volume 1

- Title 2: Inderbir Singh's Textbook of Anatomy, 6th edition, Volume 2
- Title 3: Inderbir Singh's Textbook of Anatomy, 6th edition, Volume 3
- Title 4: Human Embryology by Inderbir Singh, 10th edition
- Title 5: Inderbir Singh's Textbook of Human Histology, 7th edition

**Physiology:** Essentials of Medical Physiology by K Sembulingam and Prema Sembulingam, 6th edition

**Biochemistry:** Textbook of Biochemistry for Medical Students by DM Vasudevan, Sreekumari S and Kannan Vaidyanathan, 7th edition

**Pathology:** Textbook of Pathology by Harsh Mohan, 7th edition

**Pharmacology:** Essentials of Medical Pharmacology by KD Tripathi, 7th edition

**Microbiology and Parasitology:**

- Title 1: Essentials of Medical Microbiology by Apurba Sankar Sastry and Sandhya Bhat K, 1st edition
- Title 2: Paniker's Textbook of Medical Parasitology, 7th edition

**Forensic Medicine:**

- Title 1: The Essentials of Forensic Medicine and Toxicology by KS Narayan Reddy, 33rd edition
- Title 2: Textbook of Forensic Medicine and Toxicology by PC Dikshit, 2nd edition

**PSM:**

- Title 1: Park's Textbook of Preventive and Social Medicine by K Park, 26th edition
- Title 2: Community Medicine with Recent Advances by AH Suryakantha, 3rd edition

**ENT:** Diseases of Ear, Nose and Throat by Mohan Bansal, 1st edition

**Ophthalmology:** Comprehensive Ophthalmology by AK Khurana, Aruj K Khurana and Bhawna Khurana, 6th edition

**Medicine:**

- Title 1: Manual of Practical Medicine by R Alagappan, 5th edition
- Title 2: Textbook of Medicine by KV Krishna Das, 5th edition

**Surgery:** SRB's Manual of Surgery by Sriram Bhat M, 4th edition

**Obstetrics:** DC Dutta's Textbook of Obstetrics, 8th edition

**Gynecology:** DC Dutta's Textbook of Gynecology, 6th edition

**Dermatology:** Essentials in Dermatology, Venereology and Leprology by Ramesh Bansal, 1st edition

**Anesthesia:** Short Textbook of Anesthesia by Ajay Yadav, 4th edition

**Radiology:** Radiodiagnosis, Nuclear Medicine, Radiotherapy and Radiation Oncology by Bipin Valchandji Daga, 1st edition

**Psychiatry:** A Short Textbook of Psychiatry by Niraj Ahuja, 7th edition

**Orthopedics:** Essential Orthopedics by Maheshwari and Mhaskar, 5th edition

**Pediatrics:** Principles and Practice of Pediatrics by JN Sharma, 1st edition

# REQUEST TO READERS

With the inclination of students towards online content (Mobile Apps, YouTube etc.), there is a fall in student's interest towards printed books. I noticed that the sale of the books has fallen down to 25% (of its value in 2019). Moroever some students resort to having xerox of the books.

I will take the opportunity to request students to purchase the original books as well, otherwise authors (including me) will extinct. Save us from extinction😊.

# CONTENTS

# ANATOMY

1. **Identify the bone related to the ear:**

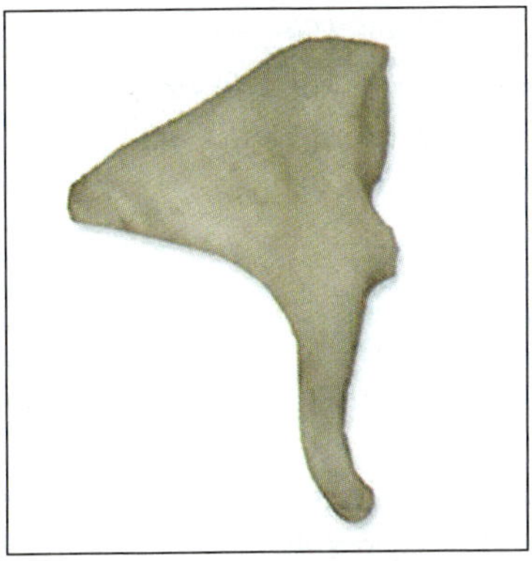

(a) Malleus (b) Incus

(c) Stapes (d) Cochlea

*Image shows incus.*

*The incus has a main part or body and two processes: long and short.*

**Ans.: B i.e., Incus**

*Reference: Page-217 (Title 3)*

2. **Which ligament is derived from the structure marked with green arrow:**

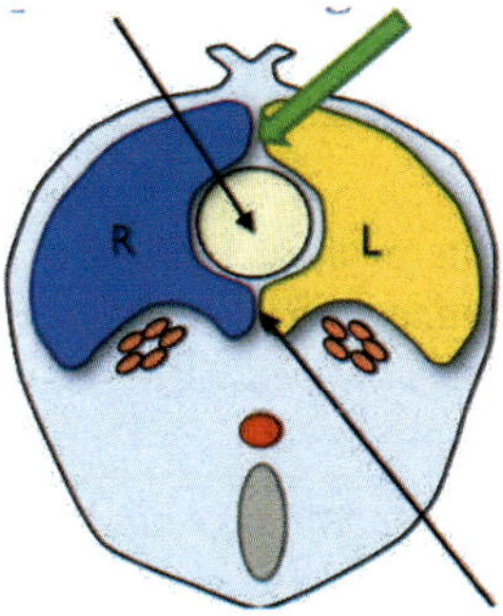

(a) Gastrosplenic ligament

(b) Gastrophrenic ligament

(c) Lineorenal ligament

(d) Falciform ligament

*Green arrow shows ventral mesogastrium/VMG.*

*It passes from the stomach to the liver, and from the liver to the diaphragm and anterior abdominal wall.*

*The part of the VMG between the liver and the stomach becomes the lesser omentum, while the part between the liver and the diaphragm (and the anterior abdominal wall) give rise to the coronary and falciform ligaments.*

**Ans.: D i.e., Falciform ligament**

***Reference: Page-186 (Title 4)***

3. **Identify the histological slide:**

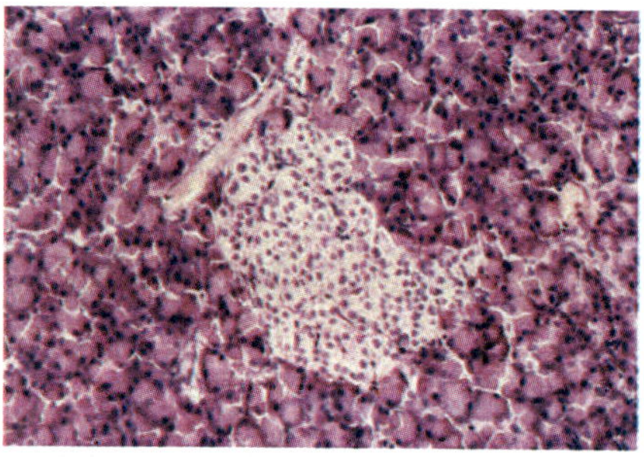

(a) Demilune

(b) Glomerulus

(c) Lymph node

(d) Islets of Langerhans

*Image shows islets of Langerhans.*

*The endocrine pancreas is in the form of numerous rounded collections of cells that are embedded within the exocrine part. These collections of cells are called the pancreatic islets, or the islets of Langerhans.*

*On microscopy, Islets of Langerhans appear as groups of small cells with lightly stained cytoplasm (as shown in the image).*

**Ans.: D i.e., Islets of Langerhans**

*Reference: Page-299, 301 (Title 5)*

**4. Identify the histological slide:**

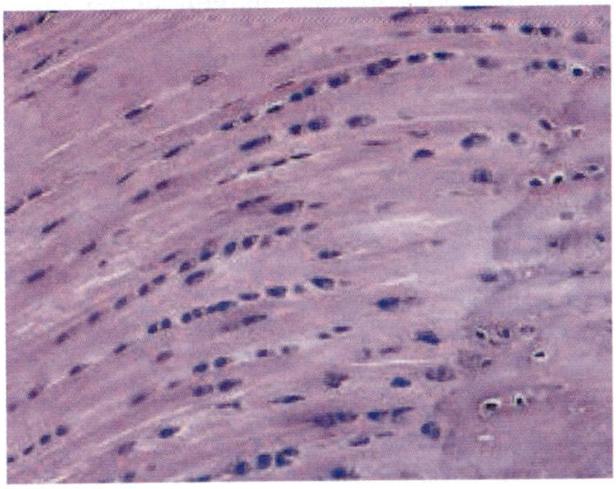

(a) Elastic cartilage (b) Fibrocartilage

(c) Hyaline cartilage (d) Bone

*Image shows fibrocartilage.*

*Fibrocartilage is characterised by presence of prominent collagen fibres arranged in bundles with rows of chondrocytes intervening between the bundles and absence of perichondrium.*

**Ans.: B i.e., Fibrocartilage**

*Reference: Page-85 (Title 5)*

# PHYSIOLOGY

**1. To promote lifespan, best recommendation is:**

(a) Reduction in calorie intake

(b) Exercise

(c) Reduce stress levels

(d) Proper sleep

*There is no direct explanation to this MCQ in the textbooks. Let us try to derive our answer from the matter given on the internet.*

*The link between calorie intake and longevity currently generates a lot of interest. Animal studies suggest that a 10–50% reduction in normal calorie intake may increase maximum lifespan.*

**Ans.: A i.e., Reduction in calorie intake**

***Reference: Internet resources***

**2. Which of the following is true regarding given cystometrogram?**

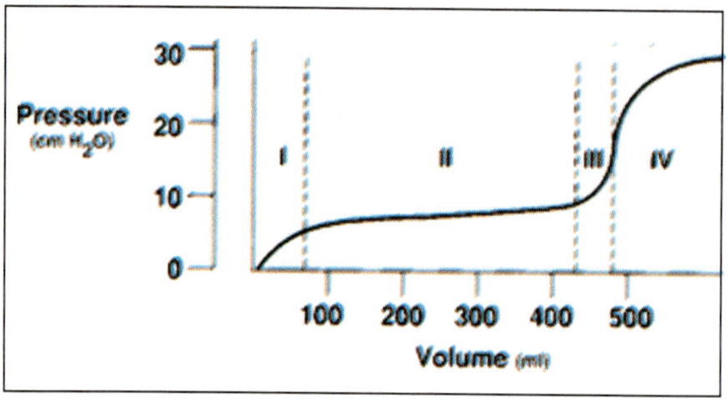


(a) Phase I denotes pressure due to residual volume

(b) Phase II is in accordance with Laplace law

(c) Voluntary control is not possible in phase III

(d) Detrusor muscle remains relaxed in phase IV

*Segment II shows the plateau, i.e., no change in intravesical pressure. It remains at 10 cm of water even after introducing 300-400 ml of fluid. It is because of adaptation of urinary bladder by relaxation.*

*It is in accordance with law of Laplace.*

*According to this law, the pressure in a spherical organ is inversely proportional to its radius, the tone remaining constant. That is, if radius is more, the pressure is less and if the radius is less, the pressure is more, provided the tone remains constant.*

$P=T/R$

*Where P is pressure, T is tension and R is radius.*

*Accordingly in the bladder, the tension increase as the urine is filled. At the same time, the radius also increases due to relaxation of detrusor muscles.*

*Because of this, the pressure does not change and the plateau appears in the graph.*

**Ans.: B i.e., Phase II is in accordance with Laplace law**

*Reference: Page-343*

3. **Extracellular concentration of potassium can be decreased by:**

(a) Lactic acid (b) Glucagon

(c) Atropine (d) Epinephrine

*There is no direct explanation to this MCQ in the textbooks. Let us try to derive our answer from the matter given on the internet.*

*Epinephrine-induced hypokalemia results from stimu-lation of a beta-adrenoceptor linked to membrane sodium/potassium adenosine triphosphatase causing potassium influx. This appears to be predominantly mediated by beta 2 receptors although beta 1 receptors may also play a part.*

**Ans.: D i.e., Epinephrine**

*Reference: Internet resources*

4. **What kind of signalling is shown in the figure?**

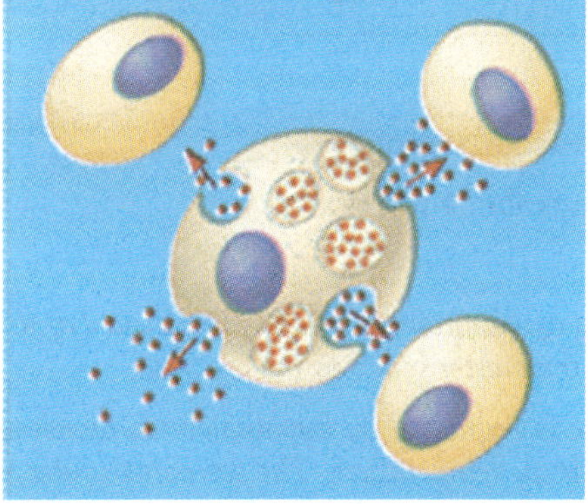

(a) Endocrine (b) Paracrine

(c) Merocrine (d) Autocrine

*Image shows paracrine signalling.*

*Paracrine messengers (red rounded structures in the image) are the chemical messengers, which diffuse from the control cells (central one in the image) to the target cells (surrounding cells in the image) through the interstitial fluid.*

**Ans.: B i.e., Paracrine**

*Reference: Page-367*

**5. Study the graph and answer the body effect, if the hypothalamic set point of temperature is raised rapidly (dotted blue line):**

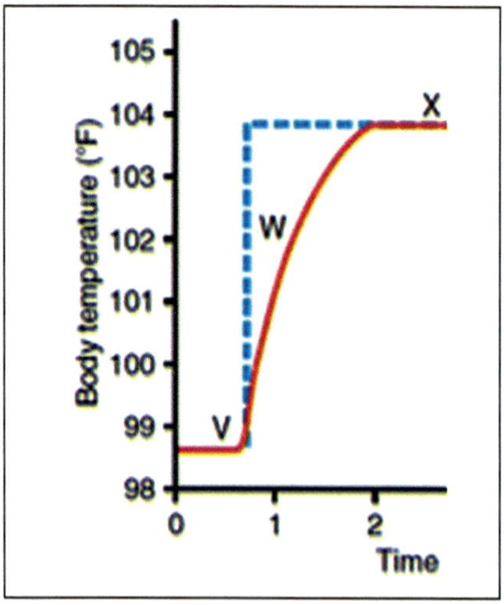


(a) Sweating

(b) Cutaneous vasodilatation

(c) Decreased metabolic reactions

(d) Shivering

*There is no direct explanation to this MCQ. Let us try to derive our answer from the matter given in the textbook.*

*Body temperature is regulated by hypothalamus, which sets the normal range of body temperature. The set point under normal physiological conditions is 98.6 degrees F.*

*When the body temperature decreases (below 98.6 degrees F), it is brought back to normal (98.6 degrees F) by 2 mechanisms: prevention of heat loss (by cutaneous vasoconstriction) and promotion of heat production (by shivering, increased metabolic reactions).*

*Now suppose (as per the MCQ) if the new set-point is made to 104 degrees F (as shown in the graph by blue dotted line), then 98.6 degrees F would be considered as a low temperature (although this is the normal value in resting conditions) and hence body will try to achieve this value (104 degrees F) from the current value (98.6 degrees F) by preventing of heat loss (by vasoconstriction) and by increasing the body temperature (by shivering and increased metabolic reactions) so as to increase the body temperature to 104 degrees F (the new set-point).*

*Hypothalamus tries to maintain the body temperature as per set-point.*

**Ans.: D i.e., Shivering**

*Reference: Page-361, 362*

**6. What kind of mechanism is involved in Baroreceptor reflex?**

(a) Feed forward

(b) Negative feedback

(c) Positive feedback

(d) Renshaw cell inhibition

*Let's discuss the baroreceptor reflex first.*

*Baroreceptors regulate the heart rate through Marey reflex.*

*Stimulation for this reflex is an increase in BP.*

*Marey reflex is a cardioinhibitory reflex that decreases the heart rate when BP increases.*

*Whenever BP increases, the aortic and carotid baroreceptors are stimulated (effectors) and stimulatory impulses are sent to the nucleus of tractus solitarius (system) via Hering nerve and aortic nerve (afferent nerves).*

*Now the NTS stimulates vasodilator area, which in turn increases the vagal tone, leading to decrease in HR.*

*Negative feedback is the one to which the system reacts in such a way as to arrest the change or reverse the direction of the change. After receiving a message, effectors send negative feedback signals back to the system. Now, the system stabilizes its own function and makes an attempt to maintain homeostasis.*

**Ans.: B i.e., Negative feedback**

*Reference: Page-40*

7. **A patient slept the whole night keeping his arm under his head. Next morning when he woke up, he had paresis and numbness in that upper limb. Which of the following physiological fact is true in relation to the clinical presentation?**
   (a) A fibers are more prone to pressure than C fibers
   (b) C fibers are more prone to pressure than A fibers
   (c) A fibers are more prone to hypoxia than C fibers
   (d) C fibers are more prone to hypoxia than A fibers

*A fibers are most susceptible to pressure.*

*B fibers are most susceptible to hypoxia.*

*C fibers are most susceptible to local anaesthetics.*

**Ans.: A i.e., A fibers are more prone to pressure than C fibers**

*Reference: Internet resources*

# BIOCHEMISTRY

1. **Which of the following is true regarding Warburg effect?**
   (a) Production of large number of ATPs
   (b) Makes cancer cells live longer

(c) Aerobic glycolysis with lactic acid production

(d) Reduced glucose uptake by cancer cells

*Warburg effect is related to aerobic glycolysis with lactic acid production.*

*Otto Warburg has studied glycolysis in various tissues. According to his studies, cancer cells utilize energy from glycolysis and they require less oxygen than the normal counterparts; this is called Warburg hypothesis (1923).*

*Rapidly growing tumour cells produce good quantity of lactic acid, causing high acidity in the local environment.*

*Lactate is used for gluconeogenesis by the liver; however, this needs large amount of energy. This is one of the reasons for cancer cachexia (loss of weight).*

**Ans.: C i.e., Aerobic glycolysis with lactic acid production**

***Reference: Page-114***

**2. Which of the following enzyme is deficient in McArdle's disease?**

(a) Glycogen phosphorylase

(b) Myophosphorylase

(c) Glucose-6 phosphatase

(d) Glucose-6-phosphatase dehydrogenase

*Type V glycogen storage disease/McArdle's disease is due to deficiency of Muscle phosphorylase enzyme (skeletal muscle).*

*It is characterized by exercise intolerance; accumulation of glycogen in muscles and myoglobinuria.*

**Ans.: B i.e., Myophosphorylase**

***Reference: Page-129t***

**3. A codon is mutated to a stop codon. What kind of mutation is this?**

(a) Mis-sense mutation

(b) Non-sense mutation

(c) Silent mutation

(d) Frameshift mutation

*If a codon is mutated to a stop codon, this is a non-sense (terminator codon) mutation.*

*For example, a tyrosine (codon, UAC) may be mutated to a termination codon (UAA or UAG). This leads to premature termination of the protein, and so functional activity may be destroyed, e.g., beta-thalassemia.*

**Ans.: B i.e., Non-sense mutation**

*Reference: Page-613*

**4. Which of the following is a complex-IV inhibitor:**

(a) Carbon dioxide (b) Cyanide

(c) Oligomycin (d) Dinitrophenol

*Complex IV inhibitors include carbon mono-oxide/CO (and not carbon dioxide), cyanide ($CN^-$), azide ($N_3^-$), hydrogen sulphide ($H_2S$).*

**Ans.: B i.e., Cyanide**

*Reference: Page-266t*

**5. Which of the following brings about DNA packing?**

(a) Glycoprotein (b) Histones

(c) Helicases (d) Chaperones

*DNA packing is a function of histones.*

*In higher organisms, DNA is organised inside the nucleus. Double stranded DNA is wound round histones to form nucleosomes. Chromatin is a loose term employed for a long stretch of DNA in association with histones. Chromatin is then further and further condensed to form chromosomes.*

**Ans.: B i.e., Histones**

*Reference: Page-576*

**6. Which of the following is true regarding telomere and telomerase:**

(a) They having coding sequence

(b) Telomerase activity is lost in cancer

(c) With ageing, the length of the telomere shortens gradually

(d) Telomerase promotes shortening of telomere

*Firstly, we should know what is telomere and what is telomerase.*

*DNA replication always takes place from 5′ to 3′ direction in the new strand. A small portion (about 300 nucleotides) in the 3′ ends of the parent strands could not be replicated.*

*This end piece of the chromosome is called telomere.*

*Unless there is some mechanism to replicate telomeres, the length of the chromosomes will go on reducing at each cell division. The stability of chromosome is thus lost.*

*The shortening of telomere end is prevented by an enzyme telomere terminal transferase or telomerase. It takes up this job of replication of the end piece of chromosomes.*

*Telomerase recognizes 3′ end of telomere, and then a small DNA strand is synthesized.*

*So, in physiological conditions, terminal restriction fragments from 70 years old donors are shorter than those from 20 years old ones. Thus, in old age, the telomerase activity is lost; leading to telomere shortening, chromosome instability and cell death.*

*As a general rule, cancer cells have continued presence of telomerase, and the chromosome length equilibrium is maintained, leading to continued cell division. As cancer cells have increased and persistent activity of telomerase, the cancer cells become immortal.*

**Ans.: C i.e., With ageing, the length of the telomere shortens gradually**

***Reference: Page-585***

**7. A Mediterranean person was taking primaquine and he developed hemolytic anemia. It was found that he was having G-6-PD deficiency. Which of the pathway is associated with this clinical syndrome?**

(a) Kreb's cycle (b) HMP pathway

(c) Glycolysis (d) Gluconeogenesis

*The affected pathway in G-6PD deficiency associated hemolysis is HMP shunt.*

*The first step catalyzed by glucose-6-phosphate dehydrogenase (G-6-PD) is the rate-limiting step in the HMP pathway.*

*NADPH generated as a result of HMP pathway is essential to maintain transparency of the eye lens, to prevent met-hemoglobinemia and to maintain erythrocyte membrane integrity.*

*Deficiency of G-6PD leads to drug-induced hemolytic anemia. The deficiency is manifested only when exposed to certain drugs or toxins, e.g., intake of anti-malarial drugs like primaquine. Primaquine stimulates peroxide formation inside RBC.*

*In G-6PD deficient cells, the level of NADPH is low; hence further production of peroxides will lead to cell lysis.*

**Ans.: B i.e., HMP pathway**

***Reference: Page-129, 136***

**8. Transport of fatty acids through mitochondrial membrane occurs via:**

(a) LCAT (b) Acyl carrier protein

(c) Carnitine (d) GLUT

*Transport of fatty acids/FA through mitochondrial membrane occurs via carnitine.*

*Fatty acids are activated in the cytoplasm; but beta-oxidation of FA is in mitochondria.*

*So, transport of FA through the mitochondrial membrane is essential.*

*The long chain FA acyl CoA cannot pass through the inner mitochondrial membrane. Therefore, a transporter, carnitine is involved in transfer of FA.*

**Ans.: C i.e., Carnitine**

***Reference: Page-151***

9. **A patient presented with mental retardation and cherry red spots on the retina. Most likely condition:**

(a) Krabbe's disease (b) Tay-Sachs disease

(c) Gaucher's disease (d) McArdle's disease

*Clinical presentation is indicative of Tay-Sachs disease.*

*Patient presents with mental retardation and cherry red spot in the macula.*

*There is progressive deterioration and the patient dies by the age of 3-4 years.*

**Ans.: B i.e., Tay-Sachs disease**

*Reference: Page-193t*

# PATHOLOGY

1. **Which of the following disease has got an autosomal recessive inheritance?**

(a) Achondroplasia

(b) Cystic fibrosis

(c) Familial hypercholesterolemia

(d) Huntington's chorea

*Cystic fibrosis has an autosomal recessive inheritance.*

*But the clinical features are apparent in homozygotes only.*

*It is a hereditary disorder characterized by viscid mucous secretions in all the exocrine glands of the body (mucoviscoidosis) and is associated with increased concentrations of electrolytes in the eccrine glands.*

**Ans.: B i.e., Cystic fibrosis**

*Reference: Page-631*

2. **A young person dies of COVID-19 infection. At lung autopsy, what is the significant finding?**

   (a) Hemorrhagic lung

   (b) Thick fibrin membrane lining the alveoli

   (c) Pulmonary edema

   (d) Hemosiderin laden alveolar macrophages

   *Clinical case series of patients with COVID-19 describe respiratory failure with moderate to severe hypoxemia and acute bilateral pulmonary infiltrates consistent with diagnosis of ARDS, the most severe form of acute lung injury (ALI).*

   *In ARDS, there is necrosis of alveolar epithelial cells and formation of characteristic eosinophilic hyaline membranes lining the respiratory bronchioles, alveolar ducts and the proximal alveoli.*

   *The membrane is largely composed of fibrin admixed with cell debris derived from necrotic alveolar cells.*

   **Ans.: B i.e., Thick fibrin membrane lining the alveoli**

   *Reference: Page-444*

3. **A young male presented with infertility. Semen analysis showed azoospermia. Testicular biopsy was done, the image of which is shown below. Most likely diagnosis:**

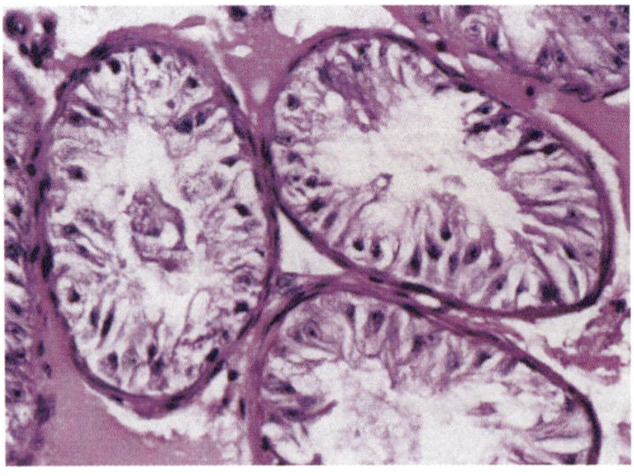

   (a) Sertoli cell–only syndrome

   (b) Orchitis

   (c) Testicular atrophy

   (d) Carcinoma of testes

*Clinical presentation and histological image are indicative of Sertoli cell–only syndrome.*

*Sertoli cell–only syndrome, also known as del Castillo syndrome or germ cell aplasia, typically occurs in males between the age of 20 and 40.*

*In this syndrome, only Sertoli cells line the seminiferous tubules of the testis (seen in the image given), and the patients have very low or absent spermatogenesis.*

**Ans.: A i.e., Sertoli cell–only syndrome**

*Reference: Internet resources*

4. **A 55 years old male presented with complaints of weakness, pallor, weight loss and a dragging sensation in the abdomen. Per abdomen examination revealed massive splenomegaly. Blood pictures showed marked leucoytosis and raised platelet count. Peripheral smear showed myelocytes and metamyelocytes. Peripheral smear image is given below. Which of the following translocation would be seen in such a case?**

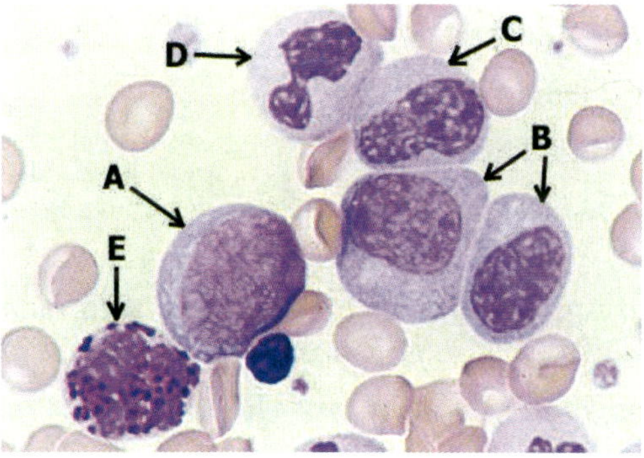


(a) t(8;14) (b) t(9;22)

(c) t(8;21) (d) t(15;17)

*Clinical presentation and histological image are indicative of chronic myeloid leukemia.*

*Clinical features of CML include features of anemia (weakness, pallor, dyspnea), symptoms of hypermetabolism (weight loss, anorexia) etc.*

*Splenomegaly is almost always present and is frequently massive.*

*Characteristically, there is marked leucocytosis (approximately 200,000/microl) or more at the time of presentation.*

*Platelet count may be normal but is raised in about half of the cases.*

*Chronic phase of CML begins as a myeloproliferative disorder and consists of excessive proliferation of myeloid cells of intermediate grade, i.e., myelocytes (marked as B) and metamyelocytes (marked as C) and mature segmented neutrophils.*

*By WHO definition, CML is established by identification of the clone of hematopoietic stem cell that possesses the balanced reciprocal translocation between chromosomes 9 and 22, forming Philadelphia chromosomes.*

**Ans.: B i.e., t(9;22)**

***Reference: Page-335, 336, 337***

**5. Rupture of saccular aneurysm results in:**

(a) Hydrocephalus

(b) Subdural hemorrhage

(c) Epidural hemorrhage

(d) Subarachnoid hemorrhage

*Rupture of a saccular aneurysm results in subarachnoid hemorrhage.*

*Berry aneurysm are saccular in appearance with rounded or lobulated bulge arising at the bifurcation of intracranial arteries.*

*They account for 95% of aneurysms which are liable to rupture.*

**Ans.: D i.e., Subarachnoid hemorrhage**

***Reference: Page-874***

**6. A patient presented with hemoglobinuria, hemosiderinuria, elevated unconjugated bilirubin and elevated LDH levels. Peripheral smear is shown below. Which of the following is related to such a condition?**

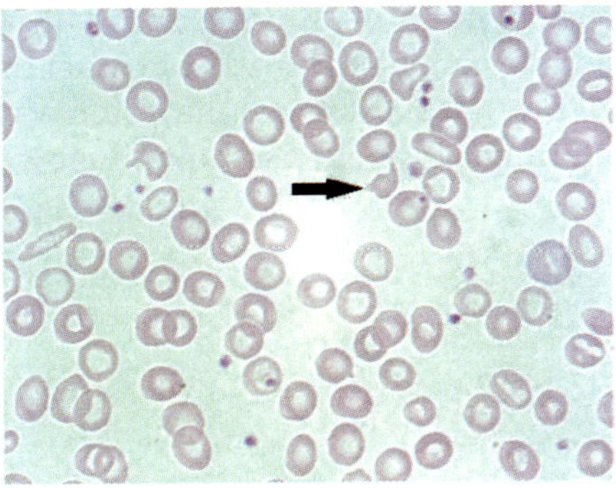

(a) Normal to high serum ferritin

(b) Splenomegaly

(c) Raised HbF

(d) Prosthetic cardiac valves

*Clinical presentation and image are indicative of microangiopathic hemolytic anemia/MAHA.*

*MAHA is caused by abnormalities in the micro-vasculature. It is generally due to mechanical trauma to the red cells in circulation and is characterized by red cell fragmentation (schistocytes, shown by black arrow in the image).*

*There are 3 different ways by which MAHA results: external impact (over bony prominences), cardiac hemolysis (prosthetic cardiac valves or artificial grafts) and fibrin deposits in microvasculature (TTP, HUS, DIC etc.).*

*MAHA comes under intravascular hemolytic anemia, in which red cell undergo lysis in the circulation and release their contents into plasma. In these cases, the plasma hemoglobin rises substantially and part of it may be excreted in the urine (haemoglobinuria).*

*Other features of intravascular hemolysis include low serum ferritin, presence of plasma hemoglobin, met-hemoglobin, hemoglobinuria and hemosiderinuria, unconjugated hyperbilirubinemia and markedly elevated serum LDH.*

**Ans.: D i.e., Prosthetic cardiac valves**

***Reference: Page-289, 290***

**7. A 40 years old white raced male presented with a slow growing small nodule on the nose medial to inner canthus of eye. Later on, it ulcerated. Biopsy of the lesion was done and the histopathological image is shown below. Most likely diagnosis:**

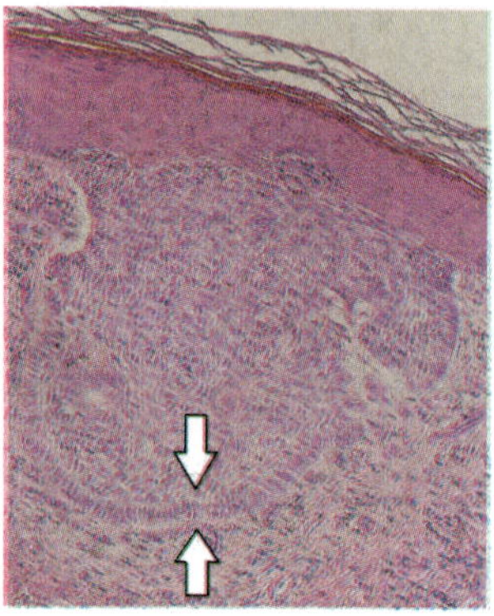

(a) Basal cell carcinoma

(b) Squamous cell carcinoma

(c) Malignant melanoma

(d) Junctional nevus

*Clinical presentation and histopathological image are indicative of Basal cell carcinoma.*

*Typically, basal cell carcinoma is a locally invasive, slow-growing tumour of the middle aged that rarely metastasises.*

*It occurs exclusively on the hairy skin, the most common location (90%) being the face, usually above the line from the lobe of the ear to the corner of the mouth.*

*Light skinned people who have little melanin is a predisposing feature.*

*Grossly, the most common pattern of BCC is a nodulo-ulcerative basal cell carcinoma in which a slow-growing small nodule undergoes central ulceration with pearly, rolled margins.*

*Histologically, the most characteristic feature is the proliferation of basaloid cells (resembling basal layer of epidermis). The most common pattern is solid basal cell carcinoma in which the dermis contains irregular masses of basaloid cells having characteristic peripheral palisaded appearance of the nuclei (white arrows in the image).*

**Ans.: A i.e., Basal cell carcinoma**

*Reference: Page-775, 776*

**8. Cystoscopic evaluation of a post-transplant patient revealed multiple soft, yellowish raised plaque in the urinary bladder mucosa. Histopathological examination of the plaque is shown in the image below. Most likely diagnosis:**

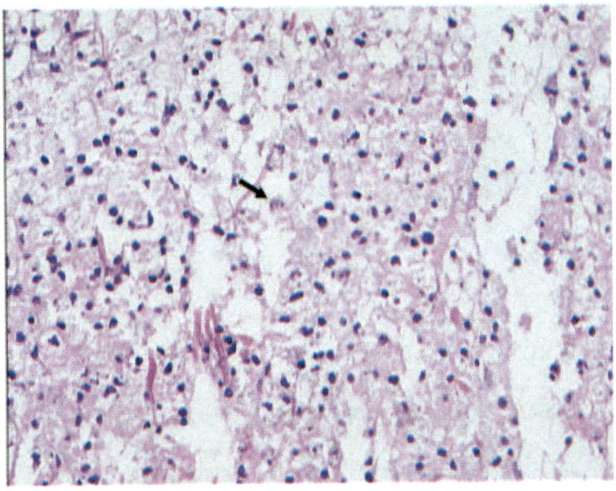

(a) Interstitial cystitis

(b) Carcinoma urinary bladder

(c) Malakoplakia

(d) Acute cystitis

*Clinical presentation and histopathological image are indicative of malakoplakia.*

*Malakoplakia occurs more commonly in immuno-suppressed patients and in recipients of transplants.*

*Grossly, the lesion appears as soft, flat, yellowish, slightly raised plaques on the bladder mucosa.*

*Microscopically, the plaques are composed of massive accumulation of foamy macrophages. These macrophages have granular PAS-positive cytoplasm and some of them contain cytoplasmic laminated concretions of calcium phosphate called Michaelis-Gutmann bodies (shown with black arrow).*

**Ans.: C i.e., Malakoplakia**

*Reference: Page-686*

9. **An adult male with history of long-standing hemorrhoids developed weakness and lethargy. Blood tests revealed a hemoglobin of 7.5 g/dl. Peripheral blood smear is shown below. Most likely diagnosis:**

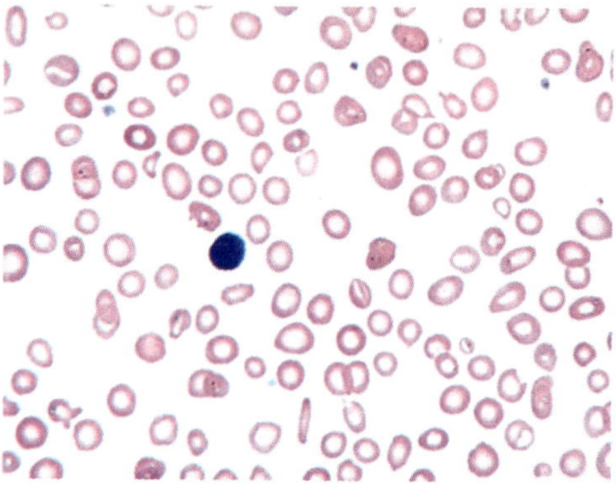

(a) Hemolytic anemia

(b) Megaloblastic anemia

(c) Iron deficiency anemia

(d) Sickle cell anemia

*Clinical presentation and peripheral blood smear are indicative of iron deficiency anemia.*

*The vast majority of cases of IDA in adult males are due to chronic blood loss.*

*Gastrointestinal tract is the usual source of bleeding which may be due to peptic ulcer, hemorrhoids, hook-worm infestation, carcinoma of stomach and large bowel, esophageal varices etc.*

*The usual symptoms of IDA are weakness, fatigue, dyspnoea on exertion, palpitations and pallor of the skin.*

*The essential feature of IDA is a fall in hemoglobin concentration up to a variable degree (normal hemoglobin in adult male: 13-18 g/dl).*

*Red blood cells in the blood film are hypochromic and microcytic (seen in the image), and there is, anisocytosis and poikilocytosis.*

**Ans.: C i.e., Iron deficiency anemia**

***Reference: Page-274, 275***

10. **What is the route of metastasis of carcinoma prostate to lumbar vertebra:**

(a) Lymphatics

(b) Prostatic venous plexus

(c) Transcoelomic spread

(d) Direct spread

*Route of metastasis of carcinoma prostate to lumbar vertebra is through prostatic venous plexus.*

*Hematogenous metastasis of carcinoma prostate most often leads to characteristic osteoblastic osseous metastases, especially to pelvis, and lumbar spine. The route of blood borne metastasis may be retrograde spread by prostatic venous plexus or via systemic circulation.*

**Ans.: B i.e., Prostatic venous plexus**

*Reference: Page-708*

11. **A young female developed a slow growing mass in the middle anterior part of the neck. After few months, she had enlargement of cervical lymph nodes on both the sides. She was subjected to biopsy and the histopathological image is shown below. Which of the following is NOT the true statement regarding this condition?**

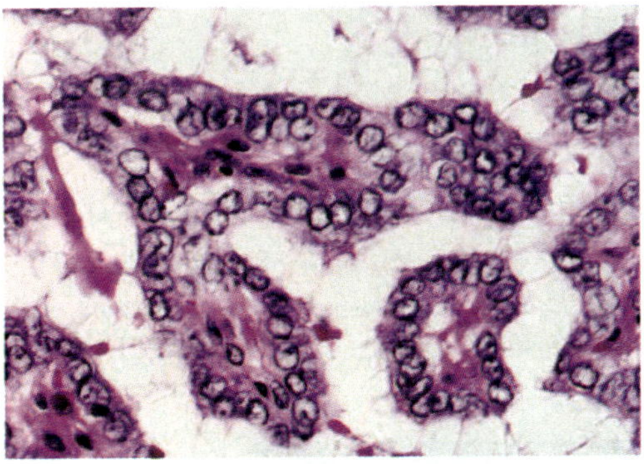

(a) Specific nuclear pattern on histology

(b) Has got good prognosis

(c) FNAC is not diagnostic

(d) Lymphatic spread is seen

*Clinical presentation and histological image are indicative of papillary carcinoma of thyroid.*

*PCT is found more commonly in young females.*

*PCT is typically a slow-growing malignant tumour, most often presenting as an asymptomatic solitary nodule.*

*Some cases first come to attention by spread to regional lymph nodes and causes cervical lymphadenopathy.*

*FNAC is the investigation of choice for PCT.*

*The tumour cells have characteristic nuclear features due to dispersed nuclear chromatin imparting it ground glass or optically clear appearance and clear or oxyphilic cytoplasm (Orphan Annie eyed nuclei as shown in the image).*

*The prognosis of PCT is good; 10-year survival rate is 80-95%, irrespective of whether the tumour is pure PCT or mixed papillary-follicular Ca.*

**Ans.: C i.e., FNAC is not diagnostic**

*Reference: Page-802, 803*

**12. Which of the following is NOT a component of MEN2B syndrome?**

(a) Marfanoid features

(b) Mucosal neuromas

(c) Megacolon

(d) Parathyroid adenoma

*Parathyroid adenoma is not a component of MEN2B.*

*MEN type 2B is the combination of medullary carcinoma of thyroid, pheochromocytoma, mucosal neuromas, intestinal ganglioneuromatosis (associated with megacolon) and marfanoid features.*

**Ans.: D i.e., Parathyroid adenoma**

*Reference: Page-819*

**13. A patient with meningitis was subjected to lumbar puncture. Gross appearance of CSF specimen is shown in**

**the first image. CSF findings were low sugar, raised protein and mononuclear leucocytosis. Most likely diagnosis:**

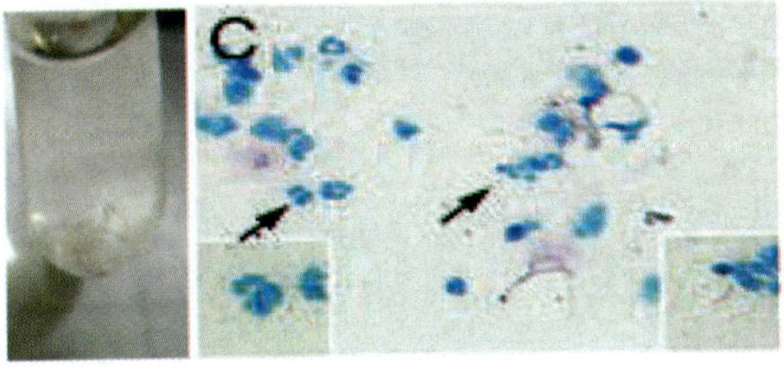


(a) Viral meningitis

(b) Acute pyogenic meningitis

(c) Tubercular meningitis

(d) Fungal meningitis

*Clinical presentation and images are indicative of tubercular meningitis.*

*Naked eye appearance of a clear or slightly turbid CSF which may for fibrin web (cob-web) on standing (1st image).*

*There is mononuclear leucocytosis consisting mostly of lymphocytes and some macrophages (100-1000 cells/microl).*

*Tubercular bacilli may be found on microscopy of centrifuged deposits by ZN staining in TBM (2nd image).*

**Ans.: C i.e., Tubercular meningitis**

***Reference: Page-868***

**14. All of the following are true regarding Neutrophil Extracellular Trap EXCEPT:**

(a) Mitochondrial DNA

(b) Seen in sepsis

(c) Related to bacteria

(d) It includes chromatin with antibacterial properties

*Neutrophil extracellular traps (NETs) are networks of extra-cellular fibers, primarily composed of DNA from neutrophils, which bind pathogens.*

*Mitochondrial DNA is the circular chromosome found inside the cellular organelles called mitochondria.*

**Ans.: A i.e., Mitochondrial DNA**

***Reference: Internet resources***

# PHARMACOLOGY

**1. MDR-TB is defined as resistance to:**

(a) Isoniazid and Rifampicin

(b) Isoniazid, Rifampicin and Fluoroquinolones

(c) Rifampicin and Streptomycin

(d) Isoniazid, Rifampicin and Kanamycin

*MDR-TB is defined as resistance to both H (isoniazid) and R (rifampicin), and may be any number of other (1st line) drug(s).*

**Ans.: A i.e., Isoniazid and Rifampicin**

***Reference: Page-775***

**2. A 50 years old male who was recently diagnosed as pulmonary TB, was started on ATT. Later on, he presented with the complaints of tingling and numbness over fingers. He is also a chronic alcoholic. This patient should be managed by starting:**

(a) Vitamin $B_1$ (b) Vitamin $B_3$

(c) Vitamin $B_6$ (d) Vitamin $B_{12}$

*Clinical presentation is indicative of INH associated neurotoxicity.*

*INH is well tolerated by most of the patients.*

*Peripheral neuritis and a variety of neurological manifestations (paresthesias, numbness, mental disturbances, rarely convulsions) are the most important dose-dependent toxic effects.*

*These are due to interference with production of the active coenzyme pyridoxal phosphate from pyridoxine, and its increased excretion in urine.*

*Pyridoxine given prophylactically (10 mg/ day) prevents the neurotoxicity even with higher doses.*

*Prophylactic pyridoxine must be given to diabetics, chronic alcoholics, malnourished, pregnant, lactating and HIV infected persons, but routine use is not mandatory.*

*INH neurotoxicity is treated by pyridoxine 100 mg/day (in the given question).*

**Ans.: C i.e., Vitamin $B_6$**

***Reference: Page-767***

**3. A known case of COPD was started on I/V theophylline after which he developed diuresis. Such an action of theophylline is mediated through which receptors?**

(a) Phosphodiesterase receptor

(b) Adenosine receptor

(c) Beta-1 adrenergic receptor

(d) Beta-2 adrenergic receptor

*Theophylline increased urine output in diuretic-dependent critically ill children and the diuretic effect may have been potentiated by concurrent use of dopamine.*

*Adenosine receptor antagonism may be a more likely mechanism for the diuretic effect of theophylline than phosphodiesterase inhibition.*

**Ans.: B i.e., Adenosine receptor**

***Reference: Internet resources***

**4. Hypolipidemic drug, which acts by inhibiting PCSK-9:**

(a) Rosuvastatin (b) Clofibrate

(c) Evolocumab (d) Ezetimibe

*There are three pharmaceutical products available in the United States that reduce* PCSK9 *activity: alirocumab, evolocumab and inclisiran.*

**Ans.: C i.e., Evolocumab**

*Reference: Internet resources*

5. **A young patient consumed 8 tablets of 0.25 mg of Digoxin and developed features of digoxin toxicity. His heart rate was 55 beats/minute and ECG showed third degree AV block. Such a patient is best managed by:**

(a) Phenytoin (b) DC shock

(c) Digoxin Fab fragment (d) Lidocaine

*For AV block and bradycardia caused due to digoxin toxicity, atropine 0.6-1.2 mg I.M. may help; otherwise, cardiac pacing is recommended. But these options are not there in the question.*

*Digoxin antibody was developed for measuring plasma concentration of digoxin by radioimmunoassay, it has been found effective in treating toxicity as well. Digoxin specific antibody cross-reacts with digitoxin also. The Fab fragment has been marketed in Europe as DIGIBIND.*

*Cardioversion by DC shock is contraindicated in digitalis toxicity because severe conduction defects may be unmasked in the digitalis intoxicated heart.*

**Ans.: C i.e., Digoxin Fab fragment**

*Reference: Page-516*

6. **A known case of depressive illness consumed large number of TCA tablets and presented to the Emergency department with altered sensorium, dryness of mouth, sweating, postural hypotension and urinary retention. ECG was done which showed wide QRS complex. Important step in management of such a patient:**

(a) DC cardioversion (b) Sodium bicarbonate

(c) Lidocaine (d) Adenosine

*Treatment of TCA side-effects is primarily supportive with gastric lavage, respiratory assistance, fluid infusion, maintenance of BP and body temperature.*

*Acidosis must be corrected by bicarbonate infusion.*

*Diazepam may be injected to control convulsions and delirium.*

*Most important is the treatment of cardiac arrhythmias, for which propranolol/ lidocaine may be used.*

*This seems a controversial question as both sodium bicarbonate and lidocaine are used in TCA overdose, but since arrhythmias may be responsible for sudden death in these patients, so administration of antiarrhythmic is an important step in management.*

*Also, correction of acidosis will automatically correct arrhythmias.*

**Ans.: B i.e., Sodium bicarbonate**

***Reference: Page-459***

**7. A female suffering from carcinoma of ovary was started on Cisplatin. Later on, she presented to the Emergency department with the complaints of several episodes of vomiting. She was given some anti-emetic drug, which resulted in the development of muscle dystonia. Which anti-emetic drug was probably given?**

(a) Ondansetron (b) Metoclopramide

(c) Scopolamine (d) Domperidone

*Metoclopramide is generally well tolerated.*

*Sedation, dizziness, loose stools, muscle dystonias (especially in children) are the main side effects.*

*Long-term use can cause parkinsonism, galactorrhoea and gynecomastia, but it should not be used to augment lactation.*

**Ans.: B i.e., Metoclopramide**

***Reference: Page-666***

**8. Which of the following is the drug of choice in over dosage of paracetamol?**

(a) Protamine sulphate (b) Flumazenil

(c) N-acetylcysteine (d) Pantoprazole

*Specific drug for paracetamol over dosage is N-acetylcysteine.*

*150 mg/kg should be infused I.V. over 15 minutes, followed by the same dose I.V. over the next 20 hours. Alternatively, 75 mg/kg can be given orally every 4-6 hours for 2-3 days.*

*It replenishes the glutathione stores of liver and prevents binding of the toxic metabolite to other cellular constituents.*

**Ans.: C i.e., N-acetylcysteine**

***Reference: Page-207***

**9. Drug which does NOT affect pleura?**

(a) Methysergide (b) Metformin

(c) Bromocriptine (d) Nitrofurantoin

*Drugs causing pleural effusion are methysergide, bromocriptine, nitrofurantoin, amiodarone, dantrolene and procarbazine.*

**Ans.: B i.e., Metformin**

***Reference: Internet resources***

**10. A patient of deep venous thrombosis was started on some anticoagulant drug, but after 5 days, he developed some lesion over the toes. Clinical image is shown below. Which of the following drug is responsible for such a presentation?**

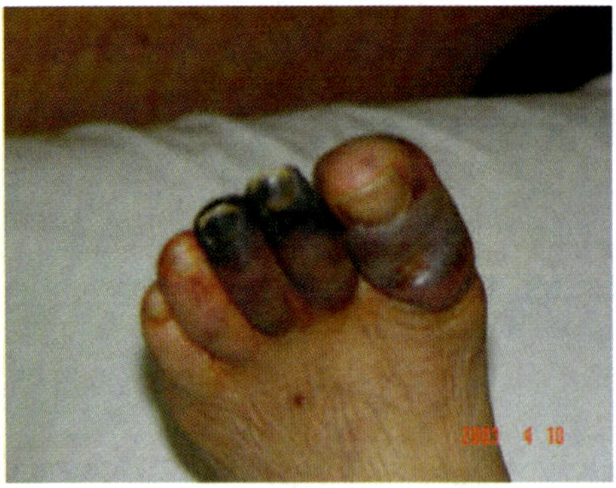

(a) Heparin (b) Warfarin

(c) Phenindione (d) Dabigatran

*Image is indicative of purple toes syndrome.*

*Purple toes syndrome is a rare adverse effect of warfarin.*

*It is characterized by a painful purple to blue discoloration of the toes.*

*The syndrome usually develops 3-8 weeks after the start of warfarin therapy.*

**Ans.: B i.e., Warfarin**

***Reference: Internet resources***

**11. A young male with urinary tract infection was given some antimicrobial agent. This agent has the tendency of causing arthropathy in children and causing tendon rupture. What is the mechanism of this antimicrobial drug given to the patient?**

(a) DNA gyrase inhibitor

(b) DHFRase inhibitor

(c) Inhibition of synthesis of mycolic acid in bacterial cell wall

(d) Inhibition of protein synthesis

*The drug discussed in the question is ciprofloxacin (prototype of fluoroquinolones/FQ).*

*Tendinitis and tendon rupture is one important adverse effect of ciprofloxacin. Risk of tendon damage is higher in patients above 60 years of age and in those receiving corticosteroids. The FQ should be stopped at the first sign of tendinitis.*

*On the basis of the finding that administered to immature pups, ciprofloxacin (and other FQ) caused cartilage damage in weight bearing joints, the FQs were contraindicated in children.*

*The FQs inhibit the enzyme bacterial DNA gyrase (primarily active in gram-negative bacteria), which nicks double stranded DNA, introduces negative supercoils and the reseals the nicked end. This is necessary to prevent excessive positive supercoiling of the strands when they separate to permit replication or transcription.*

**Ans.: A i.e., DNA gyrase inhibitor**

***Reference: Page-709***

# MICROBIOLOGY & PARASITOLOGY

1. **A patient presented with rice water stools. Which of the ganglioside receptor is affected?**
   (a) GM-1 ganglioside receptor
   (b) GM-2 ganglioside receptor
   (c) GM-3 ganglioside receptor
   (d) GD-1 alpha ganglioside receptor

   *Clinical presentation is indicative of cholera.*

   *Cholera toxin is a molecule of about 85 kDa; consists of two peptide fragments – A and B.*

   *Fragment B is the binding fragment and is pentameric, contains five subunits each weighing 11.7 kDa each. It binds to GM1 ganglioside receptors present on the intestinal epithelium, following which A fragment is internalized and cleaved into A1 and A2 peptides.*

   *Fragment A2 helps in tethering A and B subunits together.*

   *Fragment A1 is the active fragment (27 kDa), causes ADP ribosylation of G protein→upregulates the activity of adenylate cyclase→results in the intracellular accumulation of cyclic adenosine monophosphate (cAMP).*

   **Ans.: A i.e., GM-1 ganglioside receptor**

   ***Reference: Page-330 (Title 1)***

2. **Which of the following microfilaria has a sheath surrounding it and had two big nuclei at the tail tip:**
   (a) Brugia malayi (b) Wuchereria bancrofti
   (c) Onchocerca volvulus (d) Loa loa

   *The microfilariae of B. malayi, although sheathed are different in a number of respects from microfilariae bancrofti.*

*Mf. malayi is smaller in size; shows kinks and secondary curves; its cephalic space is longer; carries double stylets at the anterior end; the nuclear column appears blurred in Giemsa-stained films; and the tail tip carries 2 distinct nuclei, one terminal and the other subterminal.*

**Ans.: A i.e., Brugia malayi**

***Reference: Page-214 (Title 2)***

**3. A woodworker developed a chronic localized lesion over the legs. The lesion was irregular and cauliflower like. Histopathology of the lesion showed the presence of 'copper penny' as shown below. Most likely diagnosis:**

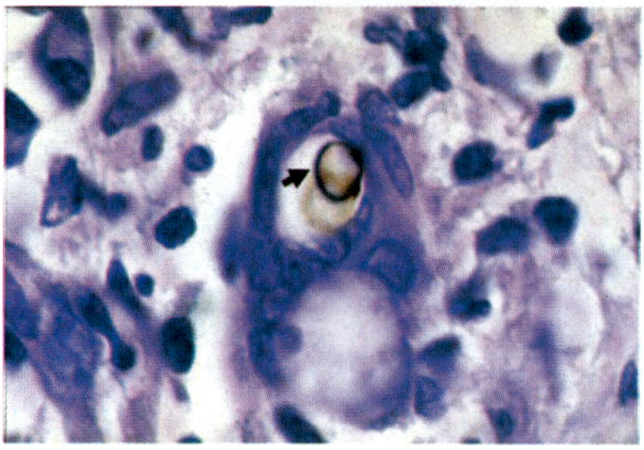

(a) Rhinosporidiosis

(b) Rhinoscleroma

(c) Chromoblastomycosis

(d) Phaeohyphomycosis

*Clinical presentation and image are indicative of chromoblastomycosis/CBM.*

*CBM refers to slow growing chronic subcutaneous lesions caused by a group of dematiaceous or phaeoid fungi (i.e., darkly pigmented fungi) that produces a characteristic morphology called sclerotic/ copper penny/medlar body (shown with the arrow).*

*Lesions in chromoblastomycosis are typically slow growing and polymorphic, such as verrucose (most common type), crusted, ulcerative and nodular or tumor like.*

*Most commonly seen in tropical or subtropical climates, often in rural areas.*

**Ans.: C i.e., Chromoblastomycosis**

*Reference: Page-561 (Title 1)*

**4. A female presented with anogenital warts. With gene study, it was found that she is having high risk HPV infection. Which will have the maximum risk?**

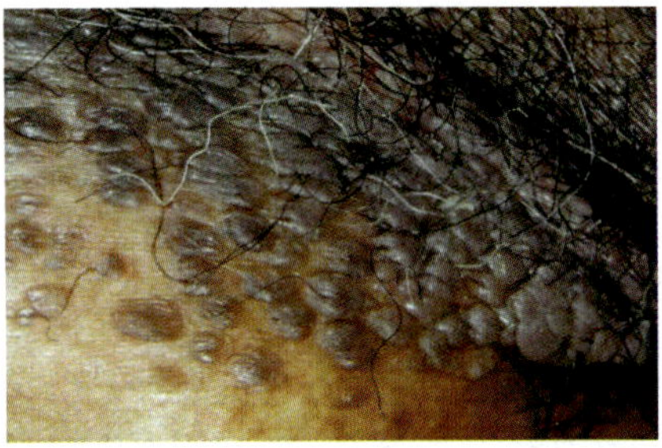

(a) HPV 6 (b) HPV 12

(c) HPV 18 (d) HPV 24

*Carcinoma of the cervix (and other genital mucosa/larynx/esophagus) have high malignant potential and the related HPV types are 16, 18, 30, 31, 33 and 45.*

**Ans.: C i.e., HPV 18**

*Reference: Page-448t (Title 1)*

**5. A farmer presented to the OPD with the complaints of multiple discharging granules from the leg. Which of the following statement is true in relation to his condition?**

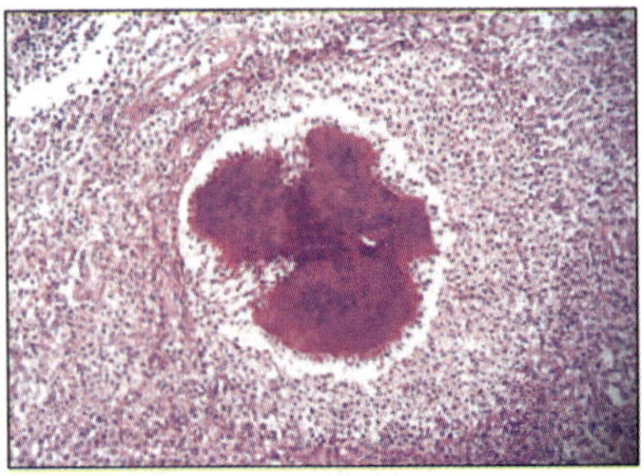

(a) Hematogenous spread

(b) Can be caused by fungi or bacteria

(c) No involvement of bone

(d) Sulfur granule contains sulfur

*Clinical presentation is indicative of mycetoma.*

*Mycetoma is a chronic granulomatous condition affecting subcutaneous tissues of the feet and hands, characterized by subcutaneous nodular swelling, multiple sinuses, discharge containing granules (shown in image) and tendency of spreading to adjacent bones (bony deformities).*

*Broadly, mycetoma is classified into two types: Eumycetoma (caused by fungi such as Madurella) and Actinomycetoma (caused by filamentous bacteria such as Nocardia, Actinomadura and Streptomyces somaliensis).*

**Ans.: B i.e., Can be caused by fungi or bacteria**

***Reference: Page-294 (Title 1)***

**6. Clostridium associated diarrhoea is best diagnosed by:**

(a) Culture of stool

(b) Culture of blood

(c) Cell culture cytotoxin test on stool

(d) PCR testing

*Let us discuss the different relevant options.*

*Stool culture is highly sensitive and specific. However, since C. difficile can colonize the GIT, only isolation is not enough to establish the infection. Toxin demonstration is more meaningful.*

*Toxin demonstration can be done by cell culture cytotoxin test on stool, enzyme immunoassay and PCR.*

*Cell culture cytotoxin test on stool is highly specific but not as sensitive as stool culture; it is time consuming.*

*PCR detecting C. difficile toxin B gene in stool – it is highly specific and sensitive.*

*Laboratory diagnosis of C. difficile infection depends on isolation of the bacilli followed by toxigenicity testing.*

*This seems a controversial question as no single choice is considered best to make a diagnosis of C. difficile infection.*

*Since we have to mark a choice, we can go with PCR testing, which is highly sensitive and specific as well.*

**Ans.: D i.e., PCR testing**

***Reference: Page-265, 266 (Title 1)***

**7. A truck driver, who is a known case of HIV-1 develops sudden onset of breathlessness, fever and lymph node enlargement. There was pleural effusion as well. His vitals were stable. Culture showed a dimorphic fungi with mold form at 25 degrees C and yeast form at 37 degrees C. Colonies show red pigmentation. What is the likely causative agent and drug used for treatment?**

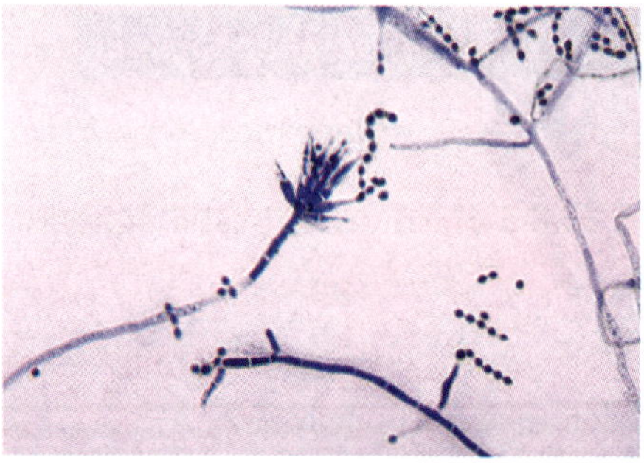

(a) Pneumocystis jirovecii, Cotrimoxazole

(b) Candida albicans, Amphotericin-B

(c) Penicillium marneffei, Amphotericin-B

(d) Aspergillus, Voriconazole

*Clinical history is indicative of Penicillium marneffei infection.*

*Penicillium/ Talaromyces marneffei affects immunocompromised hosts (e.g., patients with advanced AIDS).*

*Systemic manifestations are similar to that of disseminated histoplasmosis such as fever, weight loss, lymphadenopathy, dyspnea and hepatosplenomegaly.*

*P. marneffei being dimorphic; produces yeast like colonies at 37 degrees C and mold form at 25 degrees C in culture. The mold form has characteristic brick red pigment.*

*AIDS patient with severe penicillonisis are treated with Amphotericin-B till the condition improves followed by maintenance therapy with Itraconazole for 12 weeks.*

**Ans.: C i.e., Penicillium marneffei, Amphotericin-B**

*Reference: Page-576 (Title 1)*

8. **A patient was given intravenous botulinum toxin. What is the mechanism of action of botulinum toxin?**

   (a) Inhibits release of acetylcholine

   (b) Blockade of post-synaptic nicotinic cholinergic receptors

   (c) Inhibits reuptake of nor-epinephrine at neuromuscular junction

   (d) Inhibits degradation of acetylcholine

   *BT acts by blocking the release of Ach.*

   *After entry (either ingested, inhaled, or produced in a wound), botulinum toxin/BT is transported via blood to peripheral cholinergic nerve terminals.*

   *The most common nerve terminal sites are neuromuscular junctions, post-ganglionic parasympathetic nerve endings, and peripheral ganglia. It does not affect CNS.*

   *BT binds to acetylcholine receptors on the nerve terminals at neuromuscular junction, which results in blockage of release of acetylcholine, leading to flaccid paralysis.*

**Ans.: A i.e., Inhibits release of acetylcholine**

*Reference: Page-264 (Title 1)*

9. **A young female presented with pruritus and white curdy discharge per vaginum. Direct microscopy showed budding yeast cell with pseudo-hyphae. Which of the following is used to identify the causative organism?**

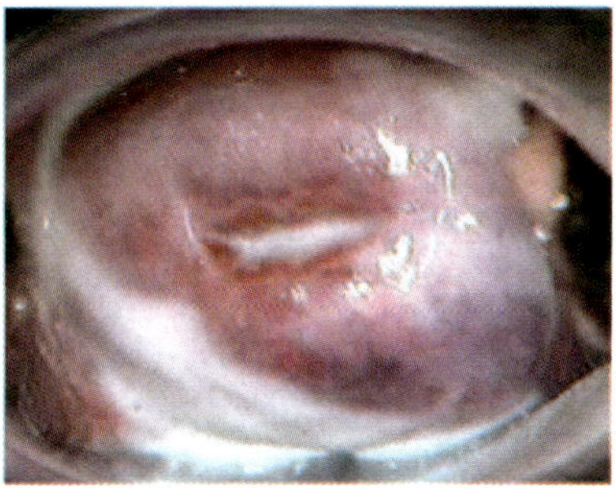

(a) Sabouraud's dextrose agar

(b) Enzyme detection methods

(c) CHROMagar

(d) Test for metabolites

*Clinical presentation is indicative of candidiasis.*

*Candidal vulvovaginitis is characterized by pruritus, pain and vaginal discharge that is usually thin, but may become whitish curd like in severe cases.*

*Candida albicans has a unique ability to transform frequently between three phenotypic forms in the tissue – yeast (blastospores), pseudohyphae and true hyphae. This is known as phenotypic switching (phenotypic dimorphism).*

*This enables adaptation to changing conditions in host and thereby assists the fungus in evading host defense system.*

*Specimens can be inoculated onto SDA with antibiotic supplements and then inoculated at 37 degrees C. Colonies of candida appear in 1-2 days and described as creamy white, smooth and pasty with typical yeasty odor.*

**Ans.: A i.e., Sabouraud's dextrose agar**

***Reference: Page-568 (Title 1)***

**10. Which of the following is considered best for diagnosing HIV infection in a baby born to an HIV infected mother?**

(a) Detection of HIV–antibodies in neonate

(b) PCR

(c) ELISA

(d) p24 antigen

*PCR detecting proviral DNA is extremely useful for diagnosis of pediatric HIV and to differentiate latent HIV infection from active viral transcription.*

*It is also useful during the window period, for viral load estimation (real time PCR) and for detection of genotypes.*

**Ans.: B i.e., PCR**

*Reference: Page-511 (Title 1)*

# FORENSIC MEDICINE & TOXICOLOGY

1. **Leading questions are permitted in:**
   (a) Cross-examination
   (b) Re-examination
   (c) Questions by the judge
   (d) Examination-in-chief

   *Leading question is one which suggests to the witness the answer desired, or which includes a material fact, and admits of a conclusive answer by a simple "Yes" or "No" (S. 141, IEA).*

   *Leading questions are permissible during cross-examination (S. 143, IEA).*

**Ans.: A i.e., Cross-examination**

*Reference: Page-14, 15 (Title 1)*

2. **A 10 years old boy presented to the Emergency department with vomiting. Parents said that he had consumed 15 tablets of ferrous sulphate. Which drug should be used in such a patient?**
   (a) d-Penicillamine (b) Dimercaprol
   (c) Desferrioxamine (d) EDTA

   *For managing iron toxicity, desferrioxamine is given.*

   *1 gm I.M. is given followed by 500 gm 4th hourly for 2 doses and finally 500 mg 4 to 12 hourly up to a maximum of 6 gm in 24 hours.*

   *It can also be given in infusion 15 mg/ kg/ hr in normal saline.*

**Ans.: C i.e., Desferrioxamine**

*Reference: Page-548 (Title 1)*

3. **A 50 years old male presented with loss of hairs of head and loss of eyebrows. His wife said that he is also having some behavioural changes. Doctor looked at the nail to reach up to the diagnosis. Poisoning is most probably due to:**

   (a) Thallium (b) Arsenic

   (c) Lead (d) Mercury

   *Clinical presentation is indicative of Thallium poisoning.*

   *Thallium triad is characterised by alopecia, skin rashes, painful peripheral neuropathy and mental confusion with lethargy.*

   *Hair loss occurs after one to two weeks. Large tufts tend to come away.*

   *Loss of outer third of eyebrows is said to be very significant.*

   *There may be Mees line on the nails.*

**Ans.: A i.e., Thallium**

*Reference: Page-548 (Title 1)*

4. **A patient presented with complaints of fatigue, constipation, headache, insomnia and joint pains. He is working in a pain factory since last 20 years. Blood test revealed anemia. Which enzyme is affected?**

   (a) Uroporphyrinogen I synthase

   (b) Uroporphyrinogen III synthase

   (c) ALA synthase

   (d) ALA dehydratase

   *Clinical presentation is indicative of lead poisoning.*

   *Features of lead poisoning include colic and constipation (dry bellyache), lead encephalopathy (insomnia, headache), anemia (fatigue) etc.*

   *Sources of chronic lead poisoning include inhalation of lead dust and fumes by persons employed in factories and industries such as painters, enamel workers etc.*

*Hemoglobin levels below 13 gm/dl are suggestive of lead poisoning.*

*Most lead poisoning symptoms are thought to occur by interfering with an essential enzyme Delta-amino-levulinic acid dehydratase, also known as PBG synthase (and also ferrochelatase).*

*So, for enzyme inhibited in lead poisoning, remember 3 names: Ferrochelatase and ALA dehydratase (also known as PBG synthase).*

**Ans.: D i.e., ALA dehydratase**

***Reference: Page-482 (Title 2)***

5. **A doctor was drunk and he performed a major surgery on a patient. Mistakenly he injured a major artery and the patient died. This is an example of:**

   (a) Dichotomy

   (b) Therapeutic misadventure

   (c) Civil negligence

   (d) Criminal negligence

   *The question of criminal negligence may arise: (1) When a doctor shows gross absence of skill or care during treatment resulting in serious injury to or death of the patient, by acts of omission or commission. (2) When a doctor performs an illegal act etc.*

**Ans.: D i.e., Criminal negligence**

***Reference: Page-40 (Title 1)***

6. **A child was brought to the hospital after burns. Calculate the burnt surface area from the image given below, as per Lund and Browder formula:**

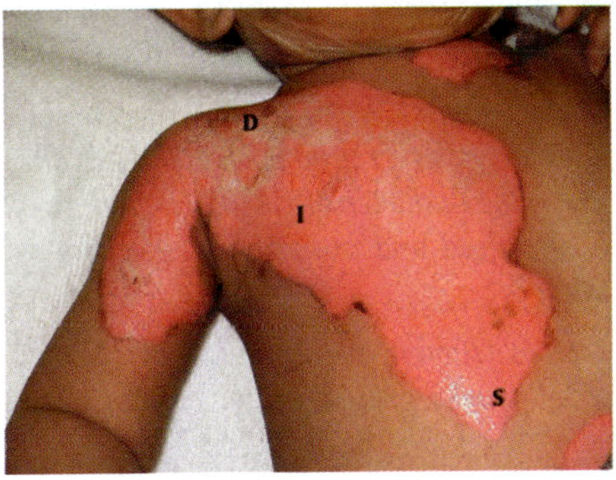

(a) 5-10% (b) 15-20%
(c) 25-30% (d) >30%

*As per Lund and Browder chart:*

*Front of trunk – one side: 6.5%*

*Front of arm – one side: 2%*

*So total burnt surface area in the given patient: 8.5%*

**Ans.: A i.e., 5-10%**

***Reference: Page-321 (Title 1)***

**7. True regarding such an injury:**

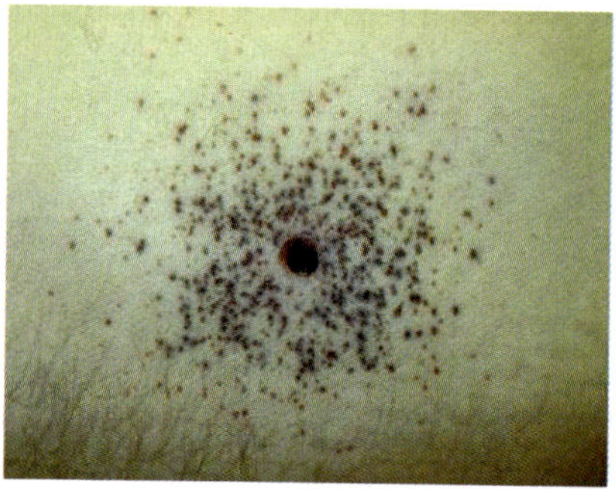

(a) Pistol, contact
(b) Pistol, near range
(c) Rifle, contact
(d) Rifle, near range

*The wound shown is by pistol, fired from a near range.*

*'Near shot' term is applied when the victim is within the range of powder deposition, and outside the range of flame and smoke, i.e., up to 50 cm.*

*The entrance wound is seen as a round hole (evident in the image), slightly smaller than the diameter of the bullet, due to elasticity of the skin, with a bruised and inverted margin and a zone of blackening and tattooing.*

*The individual tattoos (shown in the image) are caused by the individual unburned powder grains being blown into the skin.*

**Ans.: B i.e., Pistol, near range**

*Reference: Page-223 (Title 1)*

8. **Which of the statement is true regarding wound shown below?**

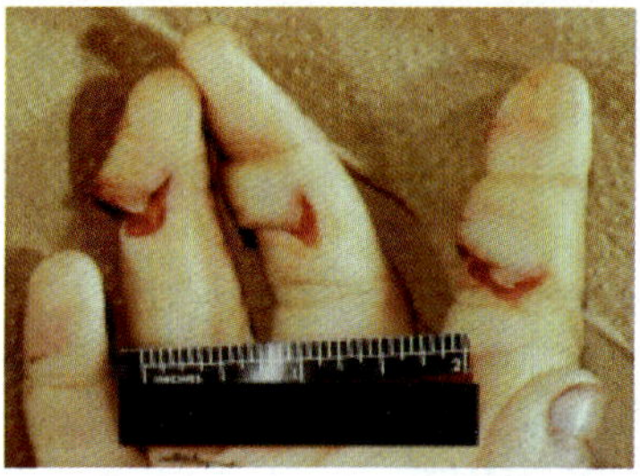

(a) Postmortem wound

(b) Suicidal wound

(c) Age of the wound is 7-8 days

(d) Defence wound

*Active defence wounds are caused when the victim tries to grasp the weapon.*

*In stabbing with a single-edged weapon, if the weapon is grasped, a single cut is produced on the palm of the hand or on the bends of the fingers or thumb (depending on the sharp side of weapon). In the image given in the question, it's on the fingers.*

*The cuts are usually irregular and ragged, because the skin tension is loosened by gripping of the knife.*

*They are often irregular in depth and distribution (as seen in the image).*

**Ans.: D i.e., Defence wound**

*Reference: Page-207 (Title 1)*

9. **A doctor explained the benefits and risks of doing a surgical procedure to the patient. After that the patient signed the consent form. This is known as:**

(a) Informed consent
(b) Implied consent
(c) Therapeutic privilege
(d) Informed refusal

*Informed consent implies an understanding by the patient of (1) The nature of his condition, (2) The nature of the proposed treatment or procedure, (3) Expectations of the recommended treatment and the likelihood of success, (4) The details of the alternative courses of the treatment that are available, (5) The risks and benefits involved in both the proposed and alternative procedure etc.*

**Ans.: A i.e., Informed consent**

*Reference: Page-51 (Title 1)*

**10. Study the given image and make a diagnosis:**

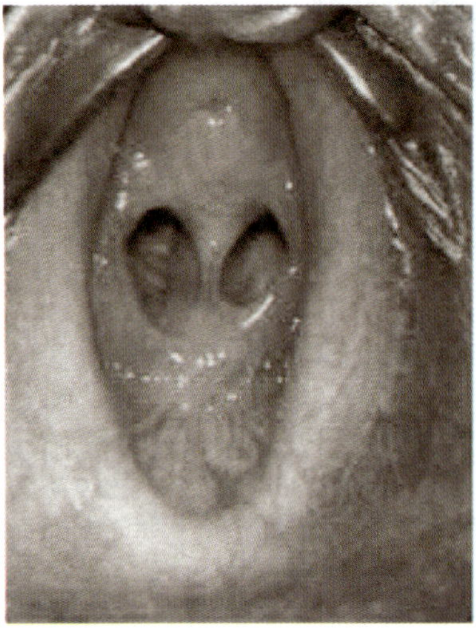

(a) Annular hymen (b) Septate hymen

(c) Imperforate hymen (d) Infantile hymen

*In septate hymen, there are two lateral openings which occur side by side, separated partially or completely by a thin strip of tissue.*

**Ans.: B i.e., Septate hymen**

*Reference: Page-390 (Title 1)*

**11. A dead body had a transverse ligature mark encircling the neck. The location was below the thyroid cartilage. There was no dribbling of saliva from the angle of mouth. This suggest:**

(a) Manual throttling

(b) Strangulation by ligature

(c) Antemortem hanging

(d) Postmortem hanging

*Presentation is indicative of strangulation by ligature.*

*The ligature mark is usually a well-defined and slightly depressed mark at any level on the neck, buy usually about the middle or below the thyroid cartilage.*

*The mark completely encircles the neck transversely, but is more prominent at the front and at the back.*

**Ans.: B i.e., Strangulation by ligature**

***Reference: Page-347 (Title 1)***

# PSM

**1. Which of the following is NOT a component of WHO STEP wise approach?**

(a) Questionnaire

(b) Biochemical measurement

(c) Psychological measurement

(d) Physical measurement

*The WHO has developed a survey methodology known as "the STEPS Non-communicable Disease Risk Factors Survey" to help countries establish non-communicable diseases/NCD surveillance system.*

*The methodology prescribes three steps – step 1: Questionnaire, step 2: Physical measurements, and step 3: Biochemical measurements.*

*The core topics covered by most surveys are demographic, health status and health behaviours.*

*These provide data on socio-economic risk factors and metabolic, nutritional and lifestyle risk factors.*

**Ans.: C i.e., Psychological measurement**

*Reference: Page-410 (Title 1)*

**2. What is true regarding an Urban CHC?**

(a) It is a referral centre for 2-3 Urban PHC

(b) Located in a city with 1.1-5 lakhs population

(c) 100 bedded facility in metro cities

(d) Set up at places where sub-district or district hospitals are not present

*Urban Community Health Centre (U-CHC) may be set up as a satellite hospital for every 4-5 U-PHCs.*

*The U-CHC would cater to a population of 2,50,000.*

*These facilities would be in addition to the existing facilities (SDH/DH) to cater to the urban population in the locality.*

*For the metro cities, the U-CHCs may be established for every 5 lakhs population with 100 beds.*

**Ans.: C i.e., 100 bedded facility in metro cities**

*Reference: Page-502 (Title 1)*

**3. You are posted at an Urban PHC. You received 1 open vial of Pentavalent vaccine and 1 open vial of MMR vaccine after 2 days of a vaccination drive. Cold chain requirements were fully met. What will you do?**

(a) Use both the vaccines

(b) Discard both the vaccines

(c) Use Pentavalent and discard MMR vaccine

(d) Use MMR and discard Pentavalent vaccine

*Open vial policy applies only to DPT, TT, Hepatitis B, Oral Polio Vaccine, Liquid Pentavalent, PCV and injectable IPV.*

*Implementation of open vial policy allows reuse of partially used multi-dose vials of applicable vaccines under UIP in subsequent session (both fixed and outreach) up to four weeks (28 days) subject to meeting certain conditions and thus reduce vaccine wastage.*

*Open vial policy does not apply to Measles/MR, BCG, Japanese Encephalitis vaccines, Rota virus.*

**Ans.: C i.e., Use Pentavalent and discard MMR vaccine**

***Reference: Page-120 (Title 1)***

4. **What is the best way to dispose broken glass injection vials?**
   (a) Red bag
   (b) Yellow bag
   (c) White container
   (d) Blue puncture proof container

   *Glassware (broken or discarded and contaminated glass including medicine vials and ampoules except those contaminated with cytotoxic wastes) and metallic body implants are discarded in cardboard boxes with blue coloured marking.*

**Ans.: D i.e., Blue puncture proof container**

***Reference: Page-887t (Title 1)***

5. **Seeds and manure supply for School Health Services under Applied Nutrition Program, were provided by:**
   (a) UNICEF (b) WHO
   (c) CARE (d) UNDP

   *UNICEF is assisting in the implementation of the Applied Nutritional Programme in the form of implements, seeds, manure and water supply equipment. Wherever land is available, the facilities provided by UNICEF should be utilized in developing school gardens.*

   *The produce may be utilized in the school feeding programmes as well as for nutrition education.*

**Ans.: A i.e., UNICEF**

***Reference: Page-665 (Title 1)***

6. **ASHA worker in the state of Madhya Pradesh motivated a lady for institutional delivery in an Urban area. Under**

**Janani Shishu Suraksha Karyakrama/JSSK, how much financial benefit would they get?**

(a) 700 to mother and 400 to ASHA

(b) 1400 to mother and 600 to ASHA

(c) 1000 to mother and 400 to ASHA

(d) 1400 to mother and 800 to ASHA

*For institutional delivery in Urban area in Low Performing State (MP, UP, Uttarakhand, Jharkhand, Bihar, Rajasthan, Chhattisgarh, Odisha, Assam and Jammu & Kashmir), mother's package is of 1000 rupees and ASHA package is of 400 rupees.*

**Ans.: C i.e., 1000 to mother and 400 to ASHA**

*Reference: Page-510t (Title 1)*

**7. Green color in triage indicates:**

(a) Dead patient
(b) Ambulatory patient
(c) Critically ill patient
(d) Moderately ill patient

*Since the health manpower resources are in shortage as compared to the casualties, the injured survivors are classified depending upon the severity of injuries and chances of survival with medical supervision. This is called as 'Triage-approach'.*

*Priority III/Green color group in triage consists of ambulatory patients of minimum risk cases.*

**Ans.: B i.e., Ambulatory patient**

*Reference: Page-883 (Title 2)*

**8. A patient was having productive cough since 4 weeks. He was diagnosed as a case of pulmonary TB and was started on ATT under National TB Elimination Program. He took all the medications timely and after completion of intensive and continuation phase, both of his sputum smear tested negative for AFB. Patient status is:**

(a) Cured
(b) Treatment completed
(c) Relapse case
(d) Treatment after default

*'Cured' refers to only new sputum smear positive patients.*

*Initially a new sputum smear positive TB patient, who has completed the treatment and has become sputum smear negative at one or one month prior to the completion of the treatment.*

**Ans.: A i.e., Cured**

*Reference: Page-364 (Title 2)*

**9. A person had a history of travelling to African country. Following his return after 3 days, he developed fever, headache, bodyache, jaundice and hemorrhagic manifestations. Despite treatment, he died. Vaccine of which of the following strain, if given prophylactically, could have saved him from dying:**

(a) Jeryl Lynn strain (b) 17-D

(c) Nakayama strain (d) Oka

*Clinical presentation is indicative of Yellow fever.*

*It is endemic only in tropical forests of Central Africa and northern part of South America.*

*Stage of infection (last for 3-4 days) is characterized by fever, headache, body ache, flushing of face, relative bradycardia (Faget's sign) etc.*

*In stage of intoxication (starts from 4th day to 5th day), jaundice develops gradually. Albuminuria and hemorrhagic manifestations are evident. There will be epistaxis, bleeding from the gums, petechial hemorrhages, later hematemesis and melena. Death supervenes within 6 to 9 days.*

*The very effective measure of protection against Yellow fever is by immunization.*

*The internationally approved vaccine for Yellow fever is 17-D vaccine.*

**Ans.: B i.e., 17-D**

*Reference: Page-443, 444 (Title 2)*

**10. Number of children from a particular community were found to have blood cancer. It was presumed that there is some chemical in the water supplied that might have caused the blood cancer. It was decided to conduct a case-**

**control study to find the association of this chemical with the occurrence of blood cancer. Children having ALL and exposed to water was taken as cases. What group of children will constitute control?**

(a) Children from the same community, not having blood cancer, not exposed to water

(b) Children from the same community, not having blood cancer, exposed to water

(c) Children from the hospital, not having blood cancer, not exposed to water

(d) Children from the hospital, not having blood cancer, exposed to water

*'Cases' is the group of persons having a particular disease under study (children with blood cancer).*

*'Controls' group should have all the features as those of cases, except that they do not have the disease under study (children without blood cancer).*

*The control group are drawn from the sources like hospital, relatives, neighbours or general population. The control group can also be selected from the same community or from the same industry or from the same school as that of cases (the best control group in this question will comprise children from the same community).*

*Study is now made by obtaining information from each member of both the groups (cases and controls), about the exposure to the suspected factor made in the hypothesis (we will ask whether they were drinking that water or not).*

*Measurement of exposure in both the groups (case and control) is done. It consists of collection of data among both cases and control groups about their exposure to the suspected cause with reference to duration and frequency of exposure (if they were drinking, then how much water per day and for how many years, they were drinking).*

*Then the 'Exposure rate' (or frequency of exposure) is calculated in both the groups (cases and controls) and compared.*

*If the exposure rate is more among the cases than among the controls, an association is said to exist between the suspected risk factor (chemical in water) and the disease (blood cancer).*

*This seems a controversial question as definition of 'Control' does not include any information about the exposure. Infact details about exposure are studied in Case-Control study.*

**Ans.: B i.e., Children from the same community, not having blood cancer, exposed to water**

*Reference: Page-254 (Title 2)*

**11. You are posted as a Medical Officer in a PHC in a seismic area. To handle emergencies, which of the following actions will you take?**

(a) Preparedness to handle any emergency

(b) Ensure resources and funds are available for quick mobilization at the time of emergency

(c) Disaster simulation programs

(d) Give instructions over loudspeakers

*Preparedness for emergency (earthquake in the given MCQ) should be in the form of money, manpower and materials.*

*It consists of the following measures: Evaluation, from the past experiences, about the risk, the area has; location of disaster-prone areas; adoption of a standard operating procedure; organization of communication, information and warning systems; development of public education program; organization of disaster simulation exercises that test response mechanisms; keeping stock of foods, drugs and other essential commodities.*

**Ans.: D i.e., Give instructions over loudspeakers**

*Reference: Page-884 (Title 2)*

**12. A 12 years old girl is suffering has clinical manifestations of rheumatic fever. She had no carditis. Which of the following is true regarding secondary prevention?**

(a) Give injection Benzathine penicillin for 5 years or until the age of 18 years, whichever is later

(b) Give injection Benzathine penicillin for 10 years or until the age of 25 years, whichever is later

(c) Give Benzathine penicillin every 3 weeks lifelong

(d) Give Benzathine penicillin only once

*'Secondary prophylaxis' is given to all the cases of Rheumatic fever to prevent rheumatic heart disease with 1.2 million units of Benzathine penicillin, once in 3 weeks, regularly for 5 years or until the age of 18 years, whichever is later. If they have developed RHD, prophylaxis is continued for life.*

**Ans.: A i.e., Give injection Benzathine penicillin for 5 years or until the age of 18 years, whichever is later**

*Reference: Page-531 (Title 2)*

**13. An army recruit presented with myalgia, fever and rashes. There were no rashes on palms and soles. Many soldiers from his battalion were found to be infested with louse. What could be the causative organism related to his clinical condition?**

(a) Rickettsia prowazekii

(b) Rickettsia typhi

(c) Rickettsia tsutsugamushi

(d) Rickettsia conorii

*Clinical presentation is indicative of epidemic typhus.*

*It is also called Louse-borne typhus.*

*It is caused by Rickettsia prowazekii, a parasite of the body louse.*

*The disease transmission is more during famine, wars, overcrowding conditions etc.*

*Clinically it is characterized by sudden onset of fever associated with headache, malaise and prostrations.*

*Macular rashes appear on 5th day, on trunk and axilla, spreads to the rest of the body sparing face, palms and soles.*

**Ans.: A i.e., Rickettsia prowazekii**

*Reference: Page-456 (Title 2)*

**14. A cohort study was undertaken to calculate the association of drinking green tea with the development of diabetes mellitus. The value for relative risk came out to be 0.86. What will be your inference?**

(a) Drinking of green tea increase chances of diabetes mellitus

(b) Drinking of green tea decreases chances of diabetes mellitus

(c) Drinking of green tea has no effect over development of diabetes mellitus

(d) Data insufficient to comment

*Relative risk/RR of 1 means there is no association (option C)*

*RR greater than 1 indicates positive association (option A)*

*RR lesser than 1 indicates negative association (option B)*

*Negative association means that the suspected factor is regarded as a protective factor.*

**Ans.: B i.e., Drinking of green tea decreases chances of diabetes mellitus**

***Reference: Page-258 (Title 2)***

**15. Which of the following is a cost-effective and rational approach for controlling Rabies in an urban area?**

(a) Testing all the dogs for Rabies

(b) Educating the general population about Rabies

(c) Removing stray dogs and vaccinating all pet-dogs

(d) Administer Rabies vaccine to the general population

*There is no direct explanation to this MCQ. Let us try to derive our answer from the matter given in the textbook.*

*Control of Rabies in dogs (and consequently in humans) can be done by elimination of all the stray, sick, dead and ownerless dogs, enforcing registration and licensing of the pet dogs, pre-exposure immunization of all pet-dogs, with a primary course of 2 TCV injections and health education of people about rabies.*

*Based on this option 'C' seems a better answer.*

**Ans.: C i.e., Removing stray dogs and vaccinating all pet-dogs**

***Reference: Page-500 (Title 2)***

**16. Average life span of women in Japan is 84 years. As Japanese population have highest life expectancy, their life expectancy statistics are used as standard in discussing premature mortality in which of the following indicator?**

(a) HALE (b) PQLI

(c) DALY (d) DFLE

*The overall burden of disease is assessed using the disability-adjusted life year (DALY), a time-based measure that combines Years of Life Lost due to premature mortality (YLLs) and years of life lost due to time lived in states of less than full health, or years of healthy life Lost due to Disability (YLDs).*

*One DALY is 'one lost year of healthy life'.*

*It is a measure of the burden of disease in a defined population and the effectiveness of the interventions.*

Ans.: C i.e., DALY

***Reference: Page-11 (Title 2)***

**17. Which of the following points are correct regarding 'At Risk' infant?**

i. Birth weight less than 2.5 kg

ii. Birth order of more than 3

iii. Single parent

iv. Artificial feeding

v. Birth weight of < 85 percentile

(a) i and ii (b) i, ii and iii

(c) i, iii and iv (d) ii, iv and v

*It is necessary to identify particularly those 'at-risk' and give them special intensive care, because it is these 'at-risk' babies that contribute so largely to perinatal, neonatal and infant mortality.*

*The basic criteria for identifying these babies include: birth weight less than 2.5 kg, birth order more than 5, working mother/single parent, artificial feeding, weight below 70% of the expected weight (i.e., II and III degrees of malnutrition) etc.*

Ans.: C i.e., i, iii and iv

***Reference: Page-617***

# ENT

**1. A young male was having his lunch in a hotel. Suddenly he started having breathlessness as shown in the figure. What should be done?**

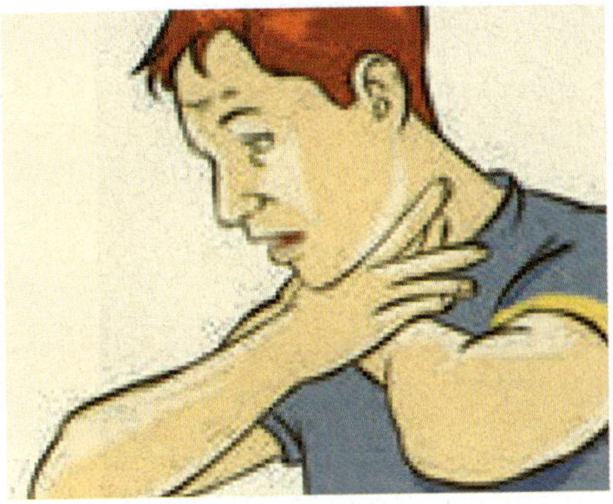

(a) Heimlich's manoeuvre

(b) Look through the mouth to see if any foreign body is there

(c) Chest thrust

(d) Back slaps

*Clinical presentation and image are indicative of foreign body/ FB (food particle in the question) in air passage.*

*Disturbed swallowing as in coughing, laughing, talking, crying or tapping on back during swallowing can result in inhalation of food into air passages.*

*During the initial period of choking (inhalational stage), gagging and wheezing is seen that lasts for some time. Small FB may be coughed out. If it is large, patient may get cyanosed and die.*

*Heimlich's manoeuvre is indicated if large bolus of food completely obstructs the larynx with total aphonia, and patient dying of asphyxia (impending death).*

**Ans.: A i.e., Heimlich's manoeuvre**

*Reference: Page-515, 516*

2. A 15 years old male presented to ENT OPD with complaints of unilateral nasal blockage and recurrent epistaxis. He is also having hearing loss. On local examination, a pink mass was seen obstructing the choana, as shown in the image below. Contrast CT scan shows enhanced uptake of contrast. Most likely diagnosis:

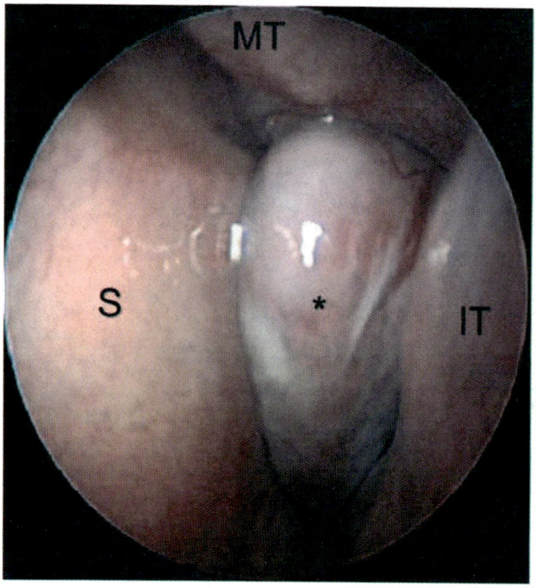


(a) Rhinosporodiosis

(b) Juvenile nasopharyngeal angiofibroma

(c) Antrochoanal polyp

(d) Foreign body

*Clinical presentation and image are indicative of juvenile nasopharyngeal angiofibroma/JNA.*

*There is profuse and recurrent episodes of epistaxis and unilateral nasal obstruction (occur in more than 80% of cases),*

*It occurs exclusively in males of 10-25 years of age.*

*Conduction hearing loss and serous otitis media occur due to obstruction of Eustachian tube.*

*There is a pink or purplish nasopharyngeal mass, which is sessile, lobulated or smooth and obstructs one or both choanae. Consistency is firm, but digital palpation is never done because it can result in profuse bleeding.*

*CT scan with contrast enhancement axial and coronal sections is the gold standard for JNA. The extent of tumor, bony destruction or displacements can be seen.*

**Ans.: B i.e., Juvenile nasopharyngeal angiofibroma**

*Reference: Page-437*

3. **A known case of asthma presented to the ENT OPD with the complaints of chronic rhinorrhoea and nasal polyps. After evaluation, a diagnosis of Samter's triad was made. Which drug should be AVOIDED in such a patient?**

(a) Aspirin (b) Co-amoxiclav

(c) Penicillin (d) Cotrimoxazole

*Samter's triad is the triad of nasal polyps, asthma and aspirin intolerance.*

**Ans.: A i.e., Aspirin**

*Reference: Page-307*

4. **A 6 years old child was brought to the ENT OPD with the complaints of hearing loss, earache and delayed speech. Otoscopic examination findings are shown below in the image. Most likely diagnosis:**

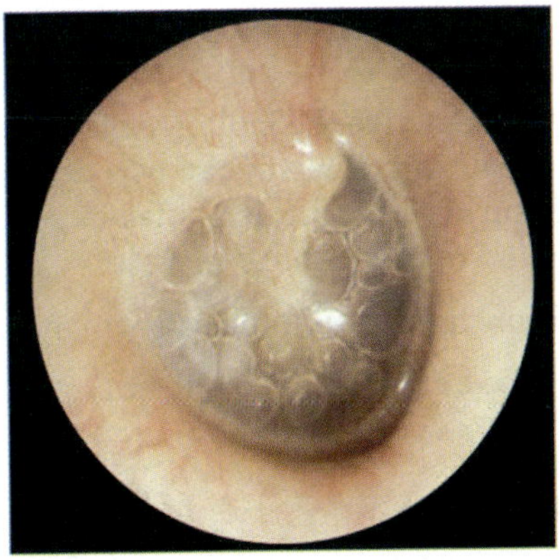

(a) Acute suppurative otitis media

(b) Chronic suppurative otitis media

(c) Otitis media with effusion

(d) Tubercular otitis media

*Clinical presentation and image are indicative of otitis media with effusion/OME.*

*In OME, there occurs collection of non-purulent nearly sterile effusion in the middle ear cleft.*

*OME may be completely asymptomatic.*

*Child turns up the volume of television and is not attentive during normal conversation.*

*Insidious conductive hearing loss (rarely exceeds 40 dB), which may be unnoticed by the parents and is accidentally discovered during audiometry.*

*Delayed and defective speech in children due to the hearing loss.*

*Mild earache.*

*Otoscopy shows retracted, less mobile or immobile tympanic membrane/TM; outward brisk movement of TM on reducing pressure in external auditory canal/ EAC with pneumatic otoscope.*

*Dark fluid filled middle ear obscures the vision of long process of incus.*

*In the image given, one can see multiple air bubbles.*

**Ans.: C i.e., Otitis media with effusion**

*Reference: Page-204*

**5. A 3 years old child presented to the Emergency department with difficulty in breathing. Chest X-ray was done and it showed hyperinflation of right side, left side being normal. True statement related to this clinical picture:**

(a) Use of flexible bronchoscope is indicated in management

(b) If there is decreased air entry on right side, it suggests foreign body

(c) Ball valve effect is the mechanism responsible for hyperinflation of right lung

(d) Clinical diagnosis is of croup is made

*Clinical presentation is indicative of bronchial foreign body.*

*Children less than 5% of age constitute more than 50% of the patients. They have the tendency to put the things in their mouth, which can go either in the food passages or air passages.*

*Right bronchus is the most common site of FBs because it is wider and more in line with the tracheal lumen. A FB may either totally obstruct a lobar/segmental bronchus (atelectasis), or produce a check valve obstruction (obstructive emphysema) which allows only ingress of air.*

*Atelectasis is due to complete step valve obstruction. It can affect lung or its segment. Poor air entry is found on auscultation of the lower lobe on the back of the thorax.*

*X-ray chest PA and lateral views especially at the end of inspiration and expiration show atelectasis and obstructive emphysema, and provide indirect evidence of radiolucent FB.*

*Rigid bronchoscopy under GA is the standard procedure for FB removal.*

**Ans.: B i.e., If there is decreased air entry on right side, it suggests foreign body**

***Reference: Page-516, 517***

**6. A patient with damage to basilar membrane presented with high frequency hearing loss. Most likely site of lesion:**

(a) Stria vascularis
(b) Helicotrema
(c) Oval window
(d) Modiolus

*Fibers near the upper end of the cochlea (i.e., helicotrema) resonate to lower frequency sound. Those near the oval window respond to higher frequencies.*

**Ans.: C i.e., Oval window**

***Reference: Internet resources***

# OPHTHALMOLOGY

1. **Which nerve is possibly involved in a person presenting with headache, lacrimation and photophobia?**

   (a) 6th CN

   (b) 5th CN

   (c) 4th CN

   (d) 3rd CN

   *There is no direct explanation to this MCQ.*

   *Since 3rd, 4th and 6th CN are concerned with ocular motility, so they can be excluded and hence 5th CN can be considered as the answer.*

   **Ans.: B i.e., 5th CN**

   *Reference: Internet resources*

2. **A patient had a history of penetrating trauma to the eye and a diagnosis of sympathetic ophthalmitis was made. Which of the following is seen?**

   (a) Pars planitis

   (b) Panuveitis

   (c) Anterior uveitis

   (d) Posterior uveitis

   *SO is a serious bilateral granulomatous panuveitis which follows a penetrating ocular trauma.*

   *The injured eye is called the exciting eye and the fellow eye which also develops uveitis is called sympathizing eye.*

   **Answer: B i.e., Panuveitis**

   *Reference: Page-437*

3. **Such a treatment is carried out for:**

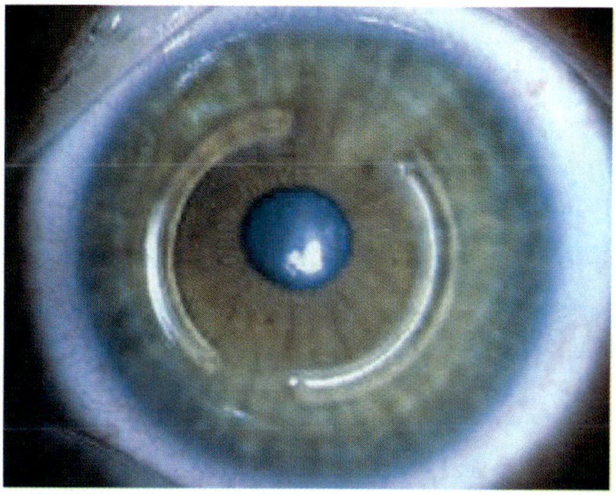

(a) Corneal dystrophy (b) Keratoconus
(c) Keratoglobus (d) High grade myopia

*INTACS, the intracorneal ring segments, are reported to be useful in early to moderate cases of keratoconus.*

**Ans.: B i.e., Keratoconus**

*Reference: Page-132*

4. **Identify the vitamin deficiency associated with the image shown below:**

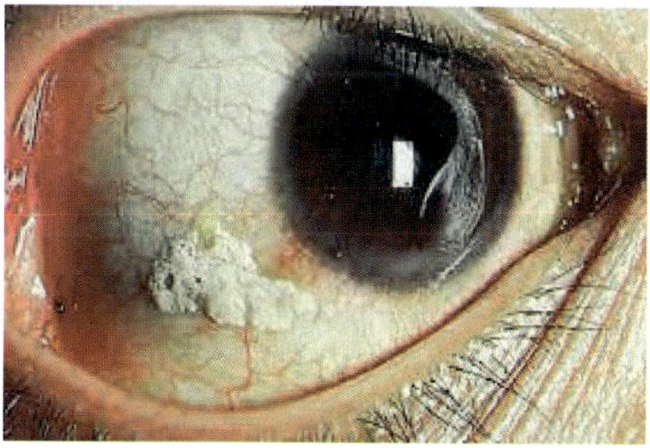

(a) Vitamin A (b) Vitamin B
(c) Vitamin C (d) Vitamin D

*Image is indicative of Bitot's spot.*

*X1B (Bitot's spots) is an extension of the xerotic process seen in stage X1A of xeropthalmia.*

*The Bitot's spot is a raised, silvery white, foamy, triangular patch of keratinized epithelium, situated on the bulbar conjunctiva in the interpalpebral area.*

*It is usually bilateral and temporal, and less frequently nasal.*

**Answer: A i.e., Vitamin A**

***Reference: Page-468***

**5. Identify the clinical condition:**

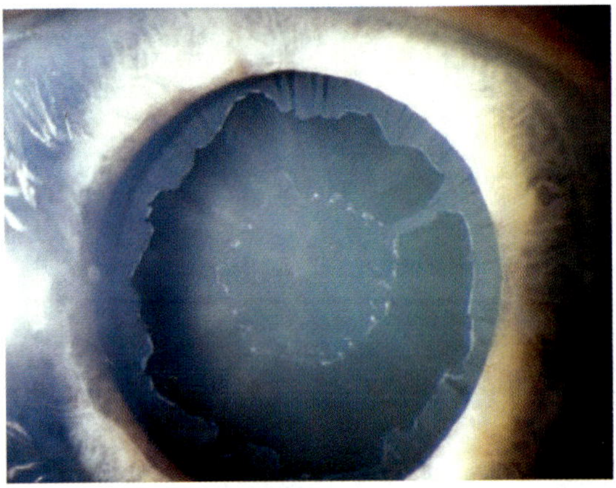

(a) Blunt trauma to eye

(b) Adherent leucoma

(c) Pseudo-exfoliation syndrome

(d) Panuveitis

*PES is characterised by deposition of an amorphous grey dandruff-like material on the pupillary border, anterior lens surface, posterior surface of iris, zonules and ciliary processes.*

**Ans.: C i.e., Pseudo-exfoliation syndrome**

***Reference: Page-250***

6. **A known case of Rheumatoid arthritis attended Ophthalmology OPD with the complaint as shown in the image below. Most likely diagnosis is:**

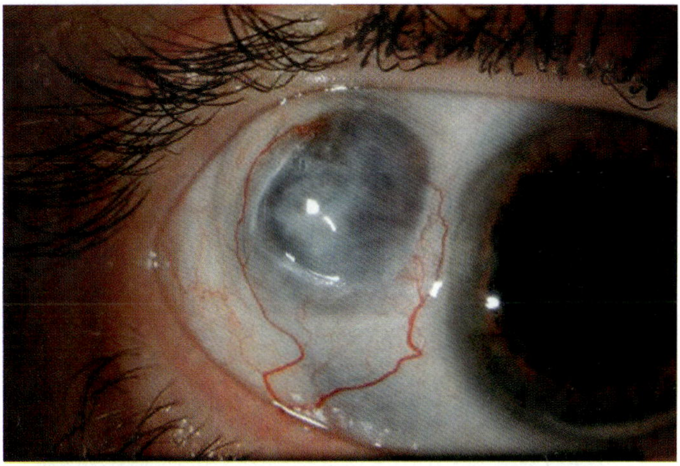

(a) Scleromalacia perforans

(b) Ciliary staphyloma

(c) Coloboma

(d) Equatorial staphyloma

*Clinical presentation and image are indicative of scleromalacia perforans.*

*Anterior necrotizing scleritis without inflammation (scleromalacia perforans) is a specific entity which typically occurs in elderly females usually suffering from long-standing rheumatoid arthritis.*

*It is characterized by development of yellowish patch of melting sclera (due to obliteration of arterial blood supply); which often together with the overlying episclera and conjunctiva completely separates from the surrounding normal sclera.*

*This sequestrum of sclera becomes dead white in colour, which eventually absorbs leaving behind it a large punched out area of thin sclera through which the uveal tissue shines.*

**Ans.: A i.e., Scleromalacia perforans**

***Reference: Page-143***

**7. A known case of diabetes mellitus had developed pre-retinal hemorrhage and neovascularization of the disc. Such a case should be managed by:**

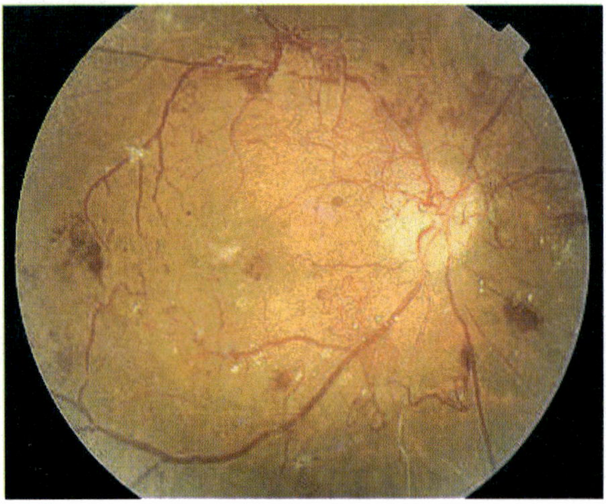

(a) Anti-VEGF drugs

(b) Grid photocoagulation by Laser

(c) Focal photocoagulation by Laser

(d) Pan-retinal photocoagulation

*Clinical presentation and image are indicative of proliferative diabetic retinopathy/PDR.*

*Occurrence of neovascularization over the changes of very severe non-proliferative diabetic retinopathy is hallmark of PDR.*

*It is characterised by proliferation of new vessels from the capillaries, in the form of neovascularization at the optic disc (NVD) and/or elsewhere (NVE) in the fundus, usually along the course of the major temporal retinal vessels.*

*NVI (Neovascularization of iris) and PDR with HRCs (high risk characteristics) are indication for PRP (pan-retinal photocoagulation).*

**Ans.: D i.e., Pan-retinal photocoagulation**

***Reference: Page-278, 281***

# MEDICINE

1. **A patient presented with a pituitary tumour with consequent overproduction of GH. He was planned for surgery but it was not possible to remove the entire tumour mass. What drug should be given to such patient to get maximum benefit?**

(a) Octreotide (b) Bromocriptine

(c) Cabergoline (d) Goserelin

*Octreotide is a synthetic analogue of somatostatin given in a dose of 50 microgram TID and is increased up to 1500 microgram/day. It produces shrinkage of the GH producing adenomas. All symptoms improve except bony changes and osteoarthritis which do not increase but can be stabilized.*

**Ans.: A i.e., Octreotide**

*Reference: Page-758, 759 (Title 1)*

2. **A 40 years old patient presented with widening of teeth gaps, protrusion of chin, prominence of frontal bone, excessive sweating, impaired glucose tolerance and enlargement of the feet and hand. Which of the following is a growth hormone receptor antagonist used to treat this condition?**

(a) Pegvisomant (b) Octreotide

(c) Cabergoline (d) Bromocriptine

*Clinical presentation is indicative of acromegaly.*

*Clinical feature of acromegaly includes soft tissue changes (skin thickening, increased sweating, enlargement of nose, lips and tongue, increased heel pad thickness etc.), acral enlargement (large hands and large feet), other bone changes (growth of lower jaw –*

*prognathism, teeth are widely spaced, skull growth – prominent supraorbital ridges with large frontal sinuses), metabolic defects (glucose intolerance, clinical DM) etc.*

*Pegvisomant is a GH antagonist that lowers IGF-1 to normal level in almost all patients.*

*The dose is 10-30 mg SC daily.*

**Ans.: A i.e., Pegvisomant**

***Reference: Page-758, 759 (Title 1)***

3. **A patient presented to the Neurology OPD with the complaints of ballistic movements of arm. He had suffered stroke 6 months back. What could be the probable site of lesion?**

(a) Putamen (b) Subthalamic nuclei

(c) Globus pallidus (d) Substantia nigra

*Clinical presentation is indicative of hemiballismus.*

*Hemiballismus is the most dramatic of all involuntary movements. It usually affects the proximal joint of one arm resulting in wild, rapid, flinging movement of wide radius, occurring constantly, interspersed with short periods of freedom. The movements may be sufficiently violent so as to injure the patient or the bystanders.*

*It is due to a lesion in the subthalamic nucleus.*

**Ans.: B i.e., Subthalamic nuclei**

***Reference: Page-631 (Title 1)***

4. **A young male was diagnosed as a case of dental caries and was planned for dental extraction procedure. All of the following conditions warrant prophylaxis for endocarditis EXCEPT:**

(a) Atrial septal defect

(b) Prosthetic heart valve

(c) Untreated cyanotic heart disease

(d) Past presentation of bacterial endocarditis

*Low or negligible risk category for IE (prophylaxis not needed): Isolated secundum ASD, surgical repair of ASD, VSD or PDA, previous coronary artery bypass graft surgery, MVP without valvular regurgitation, Physiological functional or innocent heart murmurs, cardiac pacemakers and implanted defibrillators etc.*

**Ans.: A i.e., Atrial septal defect**

*Reference: Page-804, 805 (Title 2)*

5. **An elderly male patient with coronary artery disease presented with palpitations. His blood pressure was within normal range. ECG was done which is shown below. How will you manage this patient?**

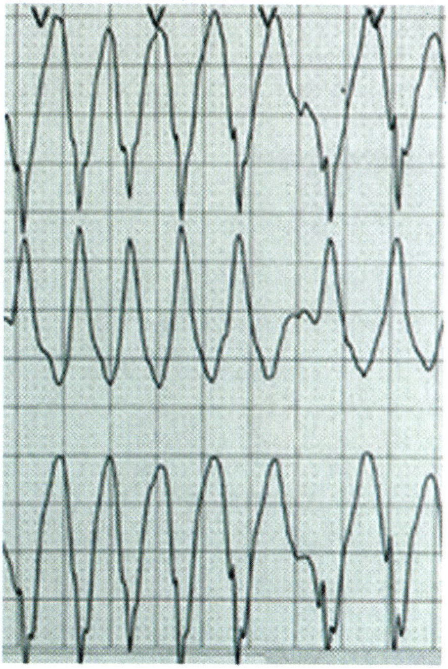

(a) Oral metoprolol

(b) Intravenous metoprolol

(c) Oral amiodarone

(d) Intravenous amiodarone

*Clinical presentation and ECG is indicative of ventricular tachycardia.*

*In uncomplicated cases, the drug of choice is lidocaine (lignocaine). It is given as a 2% solution intravenously.*

*If the VT recurs despite lignocaine, other antiarrhythmic drugs should be tried to control the arrhythmia. Drugs like procainamide disopyramide, mexiletine, propranolol or amiodarone are given intravenously for immediate control of VT.*

**Ans.: D i.e., Intravenous amiodarone**

***Reference: Page-819 (Title 2)***

6. **An elderly patient with long presentation of hypertension attended Emergency department with the complaints of acute onset of breathlessness, anxiety and sweating. It was noticed that the patient was not taking anti-hypertensives regularly. On examination, respiratory rate was 20 breaths/minute. X-ray chest was done as shown below. Next step in managing such a case:**

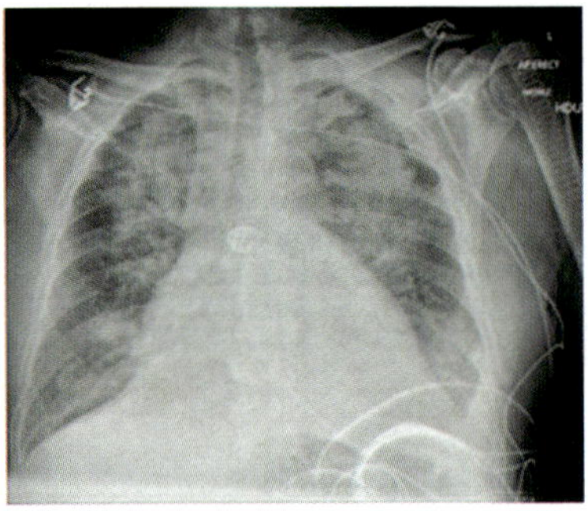

(a) Oxygen inhalation + Antibiotics

(b) Injection Nitroglycerine

(c) Injection Salbutamol

(d) Artificial ventilation

*Clinical presentation and chest X-ray is indicative of pulmonary edema.*

*One of the common causes of acute pulmonary edema is left sided heart failure (hypertensive cardiac failure).*

*Acute pulmonary edema ushers in with intense dyspnea, anxiety, and sweating. At its early phase the only obvious abnormality may be tachypnea.*

*The main steps in the treatment include the administration of oxygen, morphine, aminophylline, frusemide, digitalis and vasodilators drugs (nitroprusside, nitrates, hydralazine).*

*The patient is given oxygen immediately at a flow rate of 7-10 l/ minute.*

*Morphine allays anxiety, depress the respiratory center, allays dyspnea and reduces the adrenergic vasoconstrictor stimuli.*

*Aminophylline is very effective in increasing the cardiac output and relieving bronchospasm.*

*Option 'a' can be excluded as antibiotics are not needed in acute pulmonary edema.*

**Ans.: B i.e., Injection Nitroglycerine**

*Reference: Page-939, 940 (Title 2)*

7. **A chronic smoker presented with difficulty in breathing. His arterial blood gas analysis revealed a pH of 7.2, $pO_2$ of 70 mm Hg, $pCO_2$ of 80 mm Hg and $HCO_3$ of 34 mEq. Most likely diagnosis:**

   (a) Respiratory alkalosis

   (b) Respiratory acidosis

   (c) Metabolic alkalosis

   (d) Metabolic acidosis

   *Clinical presentation is indicative of respiratory acidosis.*

   *The arterial findings in respiratory acidosis are: $pCO_2$ is always raised (> 45 mm Hg), pH is low (< 7.35) and $HCO_3$ is high normal or slightly raised (normal is 21-30 milliequi/litre).*

**Ans.: B i.e., Respiratory acidosis**

*Reference: Page-566 (Title 1)*

8. **An elderly diabetic male presented with bloody nasal discharge and hemifacial pain on left side with loosening of a teeth from upper jaw on the left side. He is a follow-up case of COVID-19. Which of the following test would help in reaching upto a diagnosis?**

(a) MRI of head

(b) Nasal swab for mucor

(c) Glycosylated hemoglobin

(d) Serum ferritin levels

*Clinical presentation is indicative of rhinocerebral mucormycosis.*

*Rhinocerebral mucormycosis starts as sinusitis with intense headache, bloody nasal discharge, changes in mental status and black eschar of the palate (hallmark).*

*CT/MRI will reveal sinus opacification and destruction of contiguous bone with brain involvement.*

**Ans.: A i.e., MRI of head**

***Reference: Page-194 (Title 1)***

**9. A child presented to the OPD with complains of abdominal pain, vomiting and oliguria for the last 8 days. On examination he was found to be dehydrated. Serum potassium and uric acid was raised. Peripheral smear showed the presence of lymphoblasts. Immediate management of such a patient would be:**

(a) Send the child for ultrasound KUB

(b) Hydration

(c) Start Probenecid

(d) Start chemotherapy

*Clinical presentation is indicative of tumour lysis syndrome.*

*The tumour lysis syndrome is a complication of cancer chemotherapy in extensive rapidly growing and sensitive tumours due to rapid breakdown of tumour tissue. This results in the release of large quantities of cellular products into the circulation.*

*The blood concentration of uric acid, xanthine, phosphate and potassium increases very rapidly due to large scale cell destruction.*

*This condition can be prevented by good hydration in order to ensure urine flow rate of about 120 ml/ hr.*

**Ans.: B i.e., Hydration**

***Reference: Page-1146 (Title 2)***

**10. A known case of chronic liver disease with ascites had fever, abdominal pain, tenderness and reduced bowel sounds. Ascitic fluid analysis showed > 250 polymorphs/ cmm. Most likely diagnosis:**

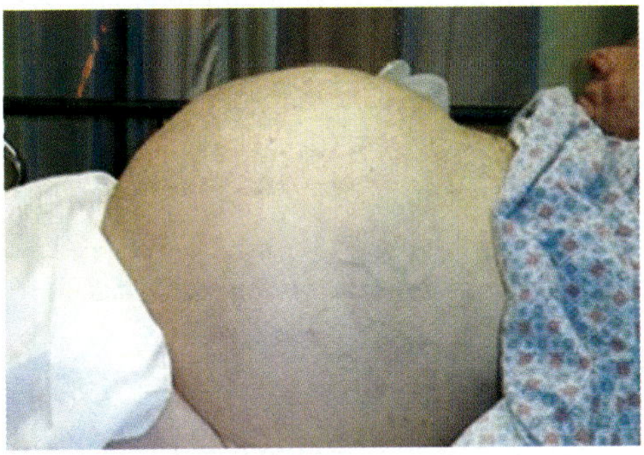

(a) Chylous ascites

(b) Spontaneous bacterial peritonitis

(c) Mucinous ascites

(d) Tubercular ascites

*Image shows ascites.*

*Criteria for diagnosis of SBP: Clinical features (fever, abdominal pain, tenderness, reduced bowel sounds and worsening of hepatic encephalopathy) + polymorphs >250/ cmm OR if polymorphs > 500/ cmm, even without clinical features.*

**Ans.: B i.e., Spontaneous bacterial peritonitis**

*Reference: Page-463 (Title 1)*

**11. A young patient presented to the Emergency with the complaint of palpitation. On palpation, pulse was weak and irregularly irregular. There was a pulse deficit of 20 beats per minute. Blood pressure was normal and heart rate was 120 beats/minute. Jugular venous pulse in this patient will show:**

(a) Canon 'a' wave

(b) Absent 'a' wave

(c) Giant 'a' wave

(d) Prominent 'v' wave

*Clinical presentation is indicative of atrial fibrillation.*

*The onset of atrial fibrillation may be felt as palpitation, especially so if the heart rate is high.*

*The pulse is totally irregular in rhythm and volume (irregularly irregular). The irregularity is best felt when the heart rate is rapid.*

*Pulse deficit can be made out by simultaneous palpation of the pulse and auscultation of the heart rate (by two different observers). A difference of more than 10 beats per minute is highly suggestive of atrial fibrillation.*

*The 'a' wave of the jugular venous pulse is abolished.*

**Ans.: B i.e., Absent 'a' wave**

***Reference: Page-821 (Title 2)***

**12. A known case of diabetes mellitus presented to the Emergency department with complaints of nausea, vomiting and abdominal pain. She is having altered sensorium. Attendants said that she never took medications regularly. General examination showed that she is dehydrated. She was having tachycardia and systolic BP was 92 mm Hg. Her serum glucose was more than 500 mg/dl. Urine showed presence of sugar and ketone bodies. Best step in managing such a case:**

(a) Intravenous fluid

(b) Insulin

(c) Intravenous fluid with regular insulin

(d) Intravenous fluid with long-acting insulin

*Clinical presentation is indicative of diabetic ketoacidosis.*

*Replacement of intravascular volume is the mainstay of treatment of DKA. Isotonic saline (0.9%) or Ringer lactate solution should be used.*

*Insulin given in a dose of 10-15 units as a bolus of 0.15 U/kg IV as an infusion is the treatment of choice in DKA.*

*Continuous infusion is given in a dose of 125 units regular insulin/250 ml NS at a rate of 0.1 unit/kg/hour (for a 60 kg individual, 6 units/hour, i.e., 5 drops/minute).*

**Ans.: C i.e., Intravenous fluid with regular insulin**

*Reference: Page-817 (Title 1)*

**13. A patient presented with fever, jaundice and calf muscle tenderness. On examination, there was conjunctival suffusion and maculopapular eruptions on the trunk. Per abdomen examination revealed tender hepatomegaly. Blood test showed thrombocytopenia and raised bilirubin level. AST and ALT are moderately raised. Kidney function test is normal. Urine microscopy showed hematuria. Most likely diagnosis:**

(a) Dengue hemorrhagic fever

(b) Fulminant hepatitis due to HAV

(c) Rickettsial disease

(d) Leptospirosis

*Clinical picture is indicative of leptospirosis.*

*Conjunctival suffusion and prominent myalgia and tenderness over big muscles are very suggestive of leptospirosis.*

*Mild thrombocytopenia may occur in up to 50% cases.*

*Bilirubin levels may exceed 30 mg/dl.*

*Aspartate (AST) and alanine aminotransferase (ALT) are moderately elevated, the elevation being considerably less compared to the rise in bilirubin. This is in contrast to the picture in viral hepatitis in which the elevation of transaminase is much more prominent.*

*Urine examination reveals proteinuria with leukocytes, erythrocytes, hyaline casts, and granular casts in the sediment.*

**Ans.: D i.e., Leptospirosis**

*Reference: Page-240, 241 (Title 2)*

**14. A patient presented with muscle weakness and polyuria. ECG showed prolonged QT interval, inverted T wave and U wave. Most likely diagnosis:**

(a) Hypokalemia

(b) Hyperkalemia

(c) Hypercalcemia

(d) Hypocalcemia

*Clinical presentation and ECG changes are indicative of hypoaklemia.*

*Hypokalemia presents as muscle weakness, ileus and polyuria.*

*ECG: 'U' wave, prolonged Q-T interval, flat or inverted T wave and premature beats.*

**Ans.: A i.e., Hypokalemia**

*Reference: Page-71 (Title 1)*

**15. An elderly patient presented with tremors, rigidity and bradykinesia. Such a patient can be treated by giving:**

(a) Haloperidol (b) Clozapine

(c) Selegiline (d) Donepezil

*Clinical presentation is indicative of Parkinson's disease.*

*Features of PD include resting tremor (usually first in fingers/thumb, coarse complex movements also known as pill rolling and drum beating movements), rigidity (seen predominantly in limbs, cogwheel type or plastic/lead pipe), hypokinesis (slowness in initiating movements) etc.*

*Selegiline and bromocriptine can be used in all ages.*

*Selegiline blocks oxidative enzymes MAO-B, it induces secretion of neurotropic factors, increase formation of oxidative enzyme superoxide dismutase, alter glutamate receptor activity etc.*

**Ans.: C i.e., Selegiline**

*Reference: Page-690, 692 (Title 1)*

**16. A young female presented with severe throbbing headache on the left side. Before the onset of headache, she had nausea, vomiting, phonophobia and photophobia. Drug which can offer her immediate relief?**

(a) Propranolol (b) Topiramate

(c) Cyproheptadine (d) Sumatriptan

*Clinical presentation is indicative of migraine with aura/classic migraine.*

*In classical migraine, the episode begins with prominent neurologic symptoms (auras) such as visual disturbances like dazzling zig-zag lines, spreading scotoma, homonymous hemianopia, field defects or rarely total blindness, sensory disturbances affecting one-half of the body, disturbances of the speech or hemiparesis.*

*These neurologic symptoms last for 15-30 minutes and usually merge into a hemi-cranial or generalized throbbing headache with nausea and vomiting, all of which may last even for 1 to 2 days.*

*Many complains of photophobia and phonophobia during the attacks.*

*Sumatriptan is effective in the treatment of acute attacks of migraine, complicated migraine or cluster headache.*

**Ans.: D i.e., Sumatriptan**

***Reference: Page-1222 (Title 2)***

**17. A 40 years old female presented with arthralgia, oral ulcers, oliguria and hematuria. Urinary examination showed the presence of RBC casts. Most likely diagnosis:**

(a) Membranous glomerulonephritis

(b) Post-streptococcal glomerulonephritis

(c) Minimal change disease

(d) Lupus nephritis

*Clinical presentation is indicative of SLE.*

*More than 60% cases are between the ages of 30 and 60.*

*Females predominate and the male to female proportion is 1:18.*

*Joint manifestation occurs in 90% of subjects with SLE in the early stages.*

*Painful ulcers may develop in the mouth and pharynx.*

*Renal involvement in SLE may remain symptomatic with only proteinuria for long intervals or may manifest as nephrotic syndrome, hematuria, acute nephritic syndrome or renal failure.*

*Acute nephritic syndrome is characterized by hematuria, red blood cells cats, proteinuria, oliguria, hypertension, fluid retention and sometimes, renal failure.*

**Ans.: D i.e., Lupus nephritis**

***Reference: Page-704 (Title 2)***

**18. A patient presented with fever and dry cough of 2 weeks duration. He is also having pain in left eye and bilateral facial weakness. His X-ray showed bilateral lymphadenopathy. Most likely diagnosis:**

(a) Lymphoma (b) Pulmonary TB

(c) Sarcoidosis (d) Carcinoma lung

*Clinical presentation is indicative of sarcoidosis.*

*General symptoms of sarcoidosis are fever, lymphadenopathy, uveoparotid fever, hypercalcemia etc.*

*Respiratory symptoms include hilar lymphadenopathy, diffuse pulmonary lesions which may be miliary, nodular or linear infiltrations, cavitations etc.*

*Nervous system symptoms include peripheral neuropathy, meningitis, cranial nerve palsies etc.*

*The most common presentation of sarcoidosis is as bilateral hilar lymphadenopathy with associated fever and erythema nodosum.*

**Ans.: C i.e., Sarcoidosis**

***Reference: Page-953 (Title 2)***

**19. A lady was on some medication for some time. Now, she is complaining of bleeding tendencies. Which vitamin deficiency is more likely in such a case?**

(a) Vitamin A (b) Vitamin D

(c) Vitamin E (d) Vitamin K

*Prolonged antibiotic therapy causes vitamin K deficiency by eliminating bacteria from the gut and consequently, reduced synthesis of vitamin K.*

**Ans.: D i.e., Vitamin K**

***Reference: Page-66***

20. **The two co-enzymes of riboflavin are FMN and FAD. Which of the following is used for evaluation of riboflavin activity?**

(a) Transketolase

(b) Glutathione reductase

(c) Hexokinase

(d) Urinary N-methyl nicotinamide

*Evaluation of riboflavin is done by RBC glutathione reductase activity.*

**Ans.: B i.e., Glutathione reductase**

*Reference: Page-74t (Title 1)*

21. **A young male presented to the OPD with complaints of drooping of the left angle of mouth, inability to blow properly and weakness of the facial muscles on the left side. Which of the following cranial nerve/CN might be paralyzed?**

(a) 4th CN (b) 5th CN

(c) 6th CN (d) 7th CN

*Clinical presentation is indicative of Bell's palsy.*

*Bell's palsy is the most common cause of unilateral LMN facial palsy.*

*The onset is abrupt with the occurrence of weakness of pursing movements of the lips, inability to hold water in the mouth, deviation of the angle of the mouth to the normal side (drooping on the affected side), incomplete closure of the eyes and watering from the eyes. While washing the oral cavity, the water escapes out of the mouth through the paralyzed side.*

**Ans.: D i.e., 7th CN**

*Reference: Page-1210 (Title 2)*

22. **A 28 years old male patient presented with the complaints of fever, malaise, jaundice, upper abdominal pain and fatigue since last 2 months. His HBV infection markers were HBsAg positive and IgM anti-HBc antibody positive. What is true?**

(a) Carrier

(b) Acute HBV infection

(c) Chronic HBV infection

(d) Recovered from HBV infection

*Clinical presentation is indicative of acute HBV infection.*

*Features of viral hepatitis are headache, fever, malaise, anorexia, distaste for cigarettes and coffee, jaundice, upper abdominal pain due to stretching of peritoneum over enlarged liver etc.*

*HBsAg appears first and is a marker of active HBV infection, appearing before the onset of symptoms and declining over 3 to 6 months.*

*Anti-HBc is usually the first antibody to appear.*

**Ans.: B i.e., Acute HBV infection**

***Reference: Page-448 (Title 1)***

**23. A 45 years old lady presented with the complaints of amenorrhoea and galactorrhoea. Her urinary pregnancy test was positive. MRI of brain revealed a large pituitary mass. She was advised surgery but she refused. Which drug is best for managing such a case?**

(a) Leuprolide (b) Bromocriptine

(c) Octreotide (d) Clozapine

*Clinical presentation is indicative of prolactinoma.*

*Prolactinomas arises from the pituitary and are the most common pituitary tumour.*

*About 50% of the patients with hyperprolactinemia develop galactorrhoea and menstrual irregularities.*

*The ratio of incidence of microadenoma (less than 10 mm in diameter) in females and males is about 20:1, while no gender difference is seen with macroadenoma (more than 10 mm in diameter).*

*CT and MRI may reveal almost all the macroadenomas.*

*MRI can detect only over 70% of the microadenomas.*

*Dopamine agonists areres the growth of the tumour, lower the secretion of prolactin and bring about clinical and biochemical relief in more than 80% of cases. Among the dopamine agonists, bromocriptine which is a derivative of ergot is most popular in India.*

**Ans.: B i.e., Bromocriptine**

***Reference: Page-615, 617 (Title 2)***

# SURGERY

1. **A child was brought to the Surgical emergency after a stab wound. His clinical picture is shown below. What is the best way to manage this patient?**

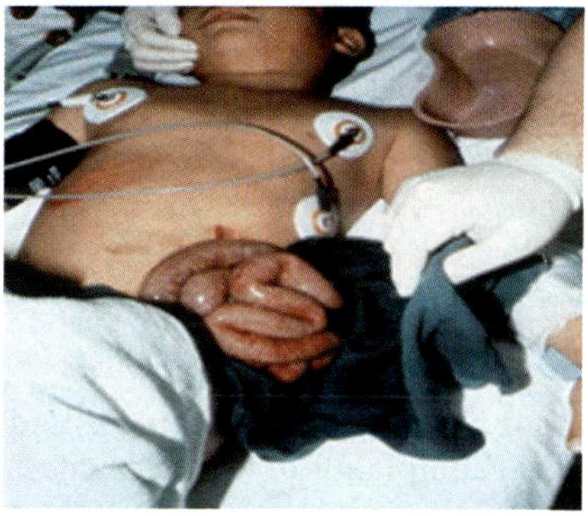

(a) Thorough debridement and closure of the wound

(b) IV fluids

(c) Exploratory laparotomy

(d) IV antibiotics for 7 days

*Clinical image is indicative of evisceration following stab injury to abdomen.*

*Abdominal stab wounds with* evisceration *remain an indication for emergency laparotomy.*

**Ans.: C i.e., Exploratory laparotomy**

***Reference: Internet resources***

2. **Study the label and identify the type of IV fluid:**

| |
|---|
| Each 100 ml contains:<br>Sodium Chloride USP 0.6 g<br>Sodium Lactate 0.31 g<br>Potassium Chloride USP 0.03 g<br>Calcium Chloride • $2H_2O$ USP 0.02 g<br>Water for injection USP qs<br>pH adjusted with HCl NF<br>pH: 6.75 (6.0-7.5)<br>Calc. Osmolarity: 275 mOsmol/liter<br>**Electrolytes (mEq/liter): $Na^+$ 130**<br>**$K^+$ 4 $Ca^{++}$ 3 $Cl^-$ 110 Lactate 28**<br>Sterile, nonpyrogenic, Single unit<br>Container. Discard unused portion.<br>Not for injection. Use only if solution is<br>clear and container and seal are intact. |

(a) Isolyte-P (b) Isoyte-M

(c) Hemaccel (d) Ringer lactate

*Ringer lactate is the most physiological fluid (crystalloid) containing sodium – 130 mEq/lt; potassium – 4 mEq/lt; chloride – 109 mEq/lt; lactate (bicarbonate) – 28 mEq/lt and calcium – 3 mEq/lt. It should be avoided in liver failure patients. As it does not contain glucose, it can be used in diabetics.*

**Ans.: D i.e., Ringer lactate**

*Reference: Page-101*

3. **A young male, who is a chronic alcoholic, presented to the Surgery OPD with the complaints of whitish patches in the oral cavity. The clinical image is shown below. Most likely diagnosis:**

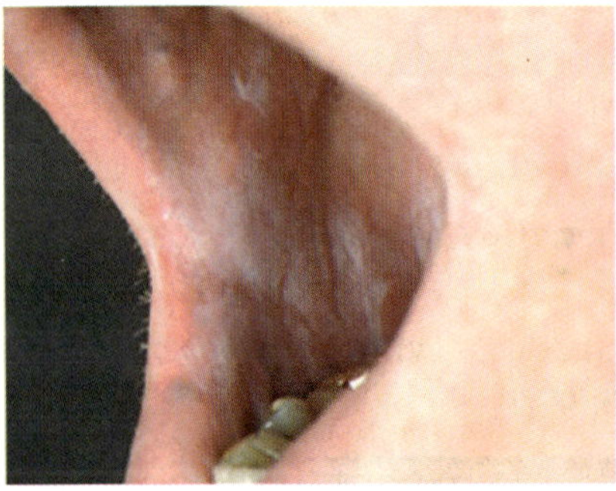

(a) Erythroplakia (b) Oral submucosal fibrosis

(c) Leukoplakia (d) Cancrum oris

*Clinical presentation and image are indicative of leukoplakia.*

*Common causes of leukoplakia are smoking, spirit, sharp tooth, sepsis, superficial glossitis, spices and pan chewing (using areca, tobacco, slaked lime).*

*Clinically the lesion appears as white or greyish coloured, well-localised patch in the cheek, tongue or palate.*

*Buccal mucosa and oral commissures are most common sites.*

*It is commoner in males (3:1).*

**Ans.: C i.e., Leukoplakia**

*Reference: Page-392*

**4. An old male presented to the Surgery OPD with the complaints of pain in the scrotum, fever and cellulitis of scrotal skin. Clinical image is shown below. Most likely diagnosis:**

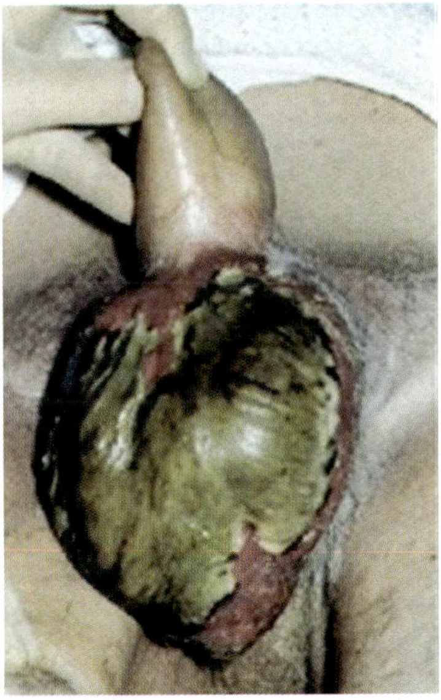

(a) Epididymo-orchitis (b) Testicular torsion

(c) Testicular carcinoma (d) Fournier's gangrene

*Clinical presentation and image are suggestive of Fournier's gangrene.*

*This condition is common in old age.*

*There is sudden pain in the scrotum, fever and severe toxicity.*

*There is very fast spreading cellulitis of scrotal skin, extending to the groin and often to anterior abdominal wall.*

*Extensive skin sloughing occurs leaving normal testis exposed.*

**Ans.: D i.e., Fournier's gangrene**

*Reference: Page-1148*

5. **A young male had a road traffic accident and presented to the Emergency with the complaint of difficulty in breathing and chest pain. Gross examination of the chest showed bruises over the chest. He was tachypneic and tachycardic. His blood pressure was 90/60 mm Hg. Chest X-ray was done as shown below. What is the best treatment of such a patient?**

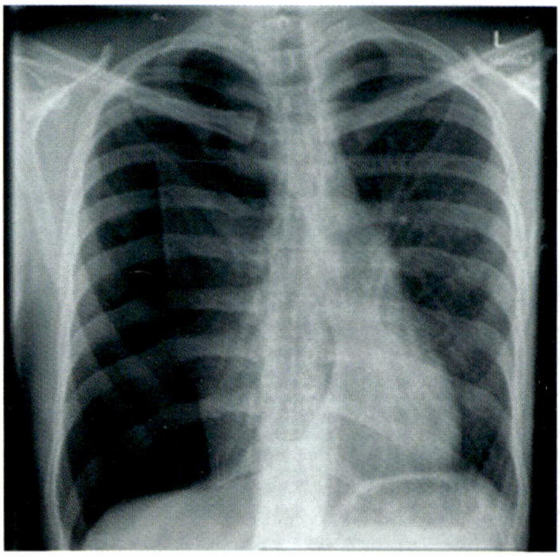

(a) Chest tube insertion and drainage

(b) Pericardiocentesis

(c) Immediate thoracotomy

(d) Ventilator assisted IPPV

*Clinical presentation and chest X-ray are indicative of tension pneumothorax.*

*Features of tension pneumothorax include tachypnea and tachycardia, decreased/absent breath sounds, resonant note on percussion with severe mediastinal/tracheal shift (seen in the given X-ray), cyanosis, hypotension and chest pain.*

*In tension pneumothorax, emergency needle aspiration is done followed by ICT (intercostal tube) placement.*

**Ans.: A i.e., Chest tube insertion and drainage**

***Reference: Page-1197***

6. **A 5 years old child presented with history of recurrent urinary tract infections. A mass was palpable in the loin as well. Micturating cystourethrogram was done, which is shown below. Most likely diagnosis:**

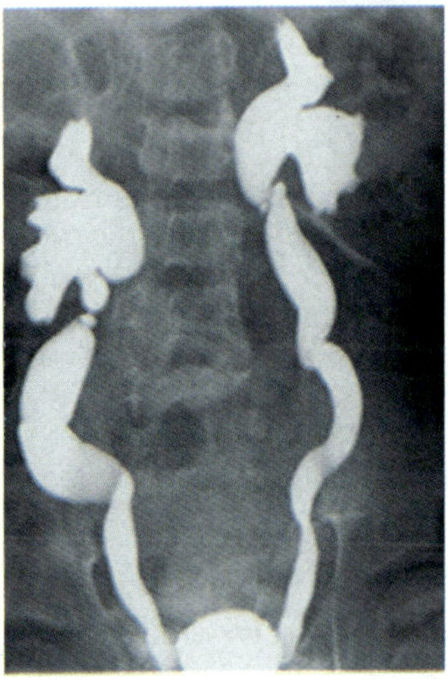

(a) Urinary bladder diverticulum

(b) Ureterocoele

(c) Vesicoureteric reflux

(d) Vesical calculi

*Clinical presentation and MCU are indicative of vesicoureteric reflux.*

*Patient presents with features of recurrent urinary tract infection and a palpable mass in the loin.*

**Ans.: C i.e., Vesicoureteric reflux**

***Reference: Page-1118***

7. **An 8 months old male child presented with sudden onset of abdominal pain with distension and vomiting. Per abdomen examination revealed a mass in right lumbar region. Attending surgeon ordered for Barium enema, which is shown below. Most likely diagnosis:**

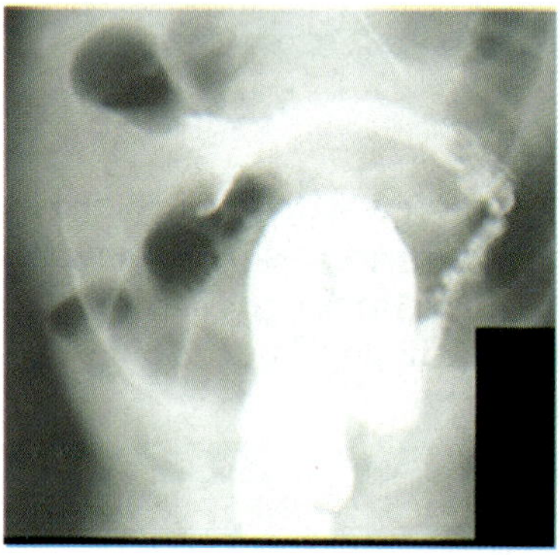

(a) Pyloric stenosis (b) Intussusception
(c) Volvulus (d) Malrotation

*Clinical presentation and Barium enema are indicative of intussusception.*

*ISS is more common in males (3:2).*

*It is common in weaning period of a child between the period of 6-9 months.*

*It is the most common cause of intestinal obstruction in infancy.*

*Initial colicky abdominal pain (75%) is present which eventually becomes severe and persistent.*

*Sudden onset of pain in a male child, with progressive distension of the abdomen, vomiting, with passage of 'red currant-jelly' stool is seen.*

*On examination, a mass is felt either on the left or on right side of the umbilicus, which is sausage shaped with concavity towards umbilicus, smooth, firm, resonant, not moving with respiration, mobile and contracts under the palpating fingers.*

*Barium enema shows a typical claw sign (seen in the image) or coiled spring sign (Pincer end).*

**Ans.: B i.e., Intussusception**

***Reference: Page-995, 996***

8. **An elderly person, who is bed ridden for many years, was having a bedsore as shown in the figure. What is the grade of this bedsore?**

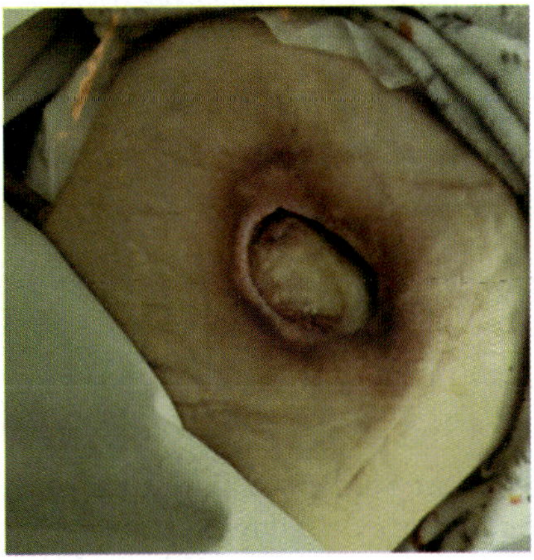

(a) Grade I (b) Grade II

(c) Grade III (d) Grade IV

*In grade IV bedsore/pressure ulcer, there is full thickness skin loss with fascia and underlying structures like muscle/ tendon/ bone etc. – Late deep ulcer.*

**Ans.: D i.e., Grade IV**

*Reference: Page-22*

9. **Amongst the following, which is the most common site of intra-abdominal abscess:**

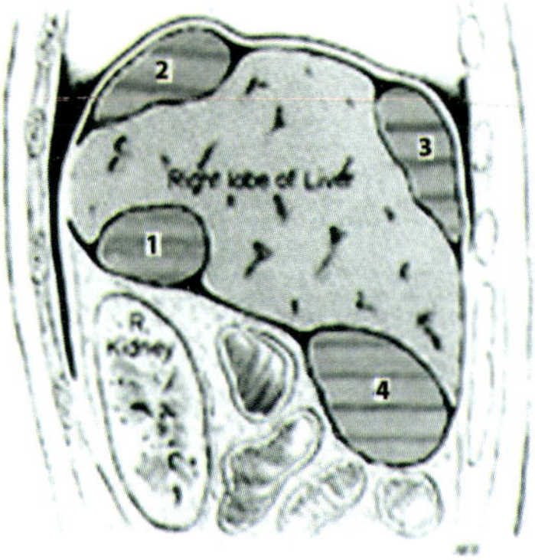

(a) 1 (b) 2

(c) 3 (d) 4

*'1' represents right posterior intraperitoneal space (right subhepatic space; Rutherford Morrison's kidney pouch).*

*It is large and deepest of all subphrenic spaces.*

*It is the most common site of subphrenic abscess.*

*Subphrenic abscess is the second most common type of intra-abdominal abscess, first being the pelvic abscess.*

**Ans.: A i.e., 1**

*Reference: Page-609*

**10. A patient presented to the Surgery OPD with the complaints of a swelling in the supraclavicular region on the right side. The swelling was smooth, compressible and pulsatile. Clinical image is given below. Next step in evaluating such a case:**

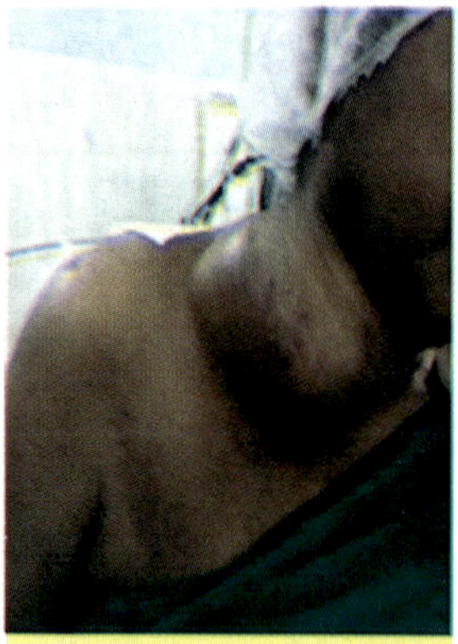

(a) CT angiography + intervention

(b) USG Doppler study

(c) Needle biopsy

(d) Excision

*Clinical presentation and image are indicative of subclavian artery aneurysm.*

*Swelling is pulsatile (expansile), smooth, soft, warm, compressible, with thrill on palpation and bruit on auscultation.*

*Swelling reduces in size when pressed proximally.*

*Investigations include Doppler study, duplex scan, angiogram, DSA (digital subtraction angiography).*

**Ans.: B i.e., USG Doppler study**

*Reference: Page-203*

**11. A male patient came to the Surgery OPD with the complaints of claudication in buttocks, thigh and calves on both the sides. Distal arterial pulses were absent. He is having impotence also. Clinical image is shown below. Most likely level of obstruction:**

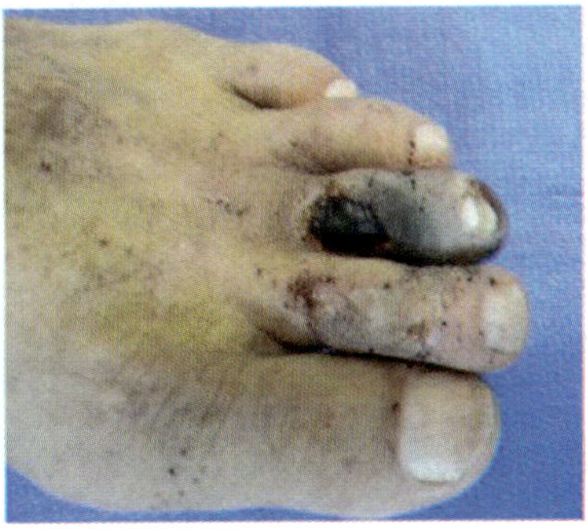

(a) Bilateral popliteal artery

(b) Bilateral femoral artery

(c) Bilateral internal iliac artery

(d) Aorto-iliac bifurcation

*Clinical presentation and image are indicative of block at the aorto-iliac bifurcation.*

*Aorto-iliac block causes claudication in both buttocks, thighs and calves; absence of femoral and distal pulses and bruit over aorto-iliac region.*

*Impotence occurs due to defective perfusion through internal iliac arteries and so into the penis causing erectile dysfunction (Leriche syndrome).*

**Ans.: D i.e., Aorto-iliac bifurcation**

*Reference: Page-178*

12. **A 40 years old patient with thyroid carcinoma underwent thyroidectomy but on 4th post-operative day, he developed perioral tingling and carpo-pedal spasm. How to investigate this patient?**

   (a) Estimation of $T_3$ and $T_4$

   (b) Radioisotope iodine scan

   (c) Estimation of calcium, phosphate and parathormone

   (d) Thyroglobulin estimation

   *Clinical presentation is indicative of hypocalcemia.*

   *Hypoparathyroidism is a rare complication of thyroidectomy surgery.*

   *Mostly it is due to vascular spasm of parathyroid glands, occurs in 2nd to 5th post-operative day.*

   *Presents with weakness, positive Chvostek's sign, carpopedal spasm, convulsions.*

   *Serum calcium estimation is done and then 10 ml of 10% calcium gluconate is given I/V 8th hourly.*

   **Ans.: C i.e., Estimation of calcium, phosphate and parathormone**

*Reference: Page-525*

13. **A young adult male presented to the Surgery OPD with the complaints of recurrent perianal openings over the buttock region. There is history of seropurulent discharge through those openings. Clinical picture of the patient is given below. Most likely diagnosis:**

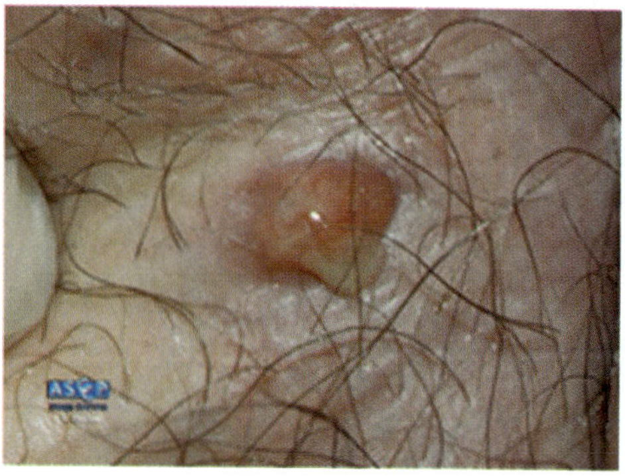

(a) Anal fissure (b) Carbuncle

(c) Pilonidal sinus (d) Fistula-in-ano

*Clinical presentation and image are indicative of fistula-in-ano.*

*It is more common in young adult males (2:1, male to female).*

*It presents with seropurulent discharge (65%), along with skin irritation and one or more external opening may be present with induration of the surrounding skin.*

*Often it may heal superficially but pus may collect beneath forming an abscess which again discharges through same or new opening. This explains its recurrent nature.*

**Ans.: D i.e., Fistula-in-ano**

***Reference: Page-1053***

**14. Study the image given below and make a clinical diagnosis:**

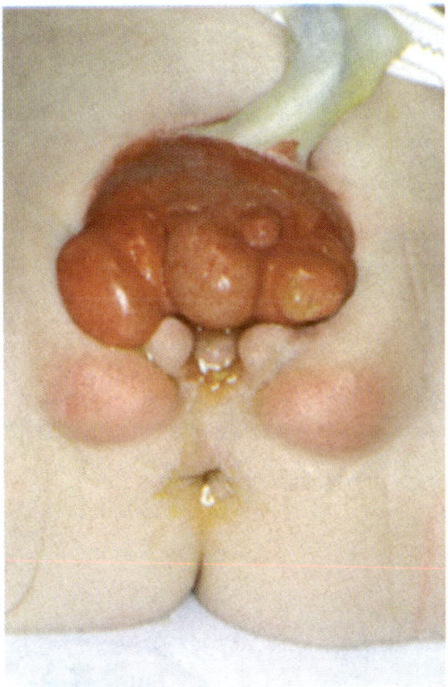

(a) Omphalocele

(b) Gastroschisis

(c) Exstrophy of the bladder

(d) Meckel's diverticulum

*Clinical image is indicative of exstrophy of the bladder/ectopia vesicae.*

*Exstrophy of the bladder is incomplete development of the infraumbilical part of the anterior abdominal wall and anterior wall of the urinary bladder.*

*Red mucus membrane of posterior bladder wall protrudes out with visible urine efflux from ureteric orifice.*

*Umbilicus is absent.*

*There is separation of pubic bones.*

**Ans.: C i.e., Exstrophy of the bladder**

***Reference: Page-1106***

**15. Study the intra-oral X-ray and make a diagnosis:**

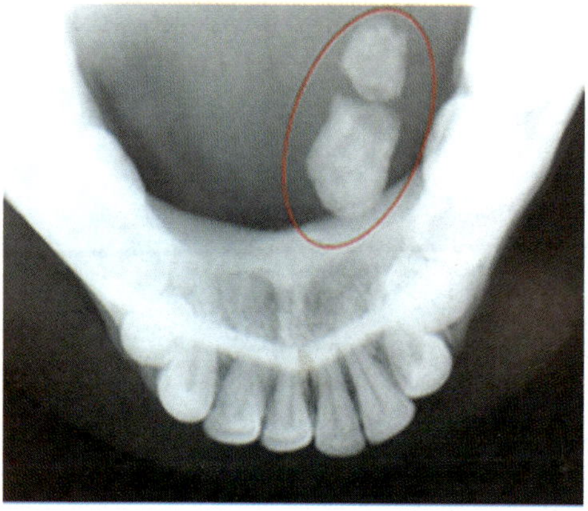

(a) Abscess in the floor of mouth

(b) Sialolithiasis

(c) Foreign body

(d) Osteoma of mandible

*Intra-oral X-ray is indicative of sialolithiasis (encircled in red).*

*Salivary calculus is seen mostly in submandibular gland duct (80%).*

*Calculi are more common in submandibular gland, because the gland secretion is viscous, contains more calcium and also, its drainage is non-dependent, causing stasis.*

*80% are radio-opaque.*

*Radiological demonstration of stone/stones is called sialolithiasis.*

**Ans.: B i.e., Sialolithiasis**

*Reference: Page-435, 436*

**16. Following stripping surgery for varicose veins, patient started complaining of numbness along the medial aspect of the thigh. This is because injury to:**

(a) Sural nerve

(b) Saphenous nerve

(c) Deep peroneal nerve

(d) Superficial peroneal nerve

*Clinical presentation is indicative of saphenous neuralgia.*

*Saphenous neuralgia (1%) is a complication of stripping of varicose vein (long saphenous vein) and occurs due to injury to saphenous nerve/avulsion.*

*It presents as numbness and tingling along especially the saphenous nerve distribution (medial aspect of leg).*

**Ans.: B i.e., Saphenous nerve**

*Reference: Page-244*

**17. A 40 years old female presented to the Surgery OPD with the complaint of lump in the breast. Clinical image of the breast is shown below. Such an appearance is because of:**

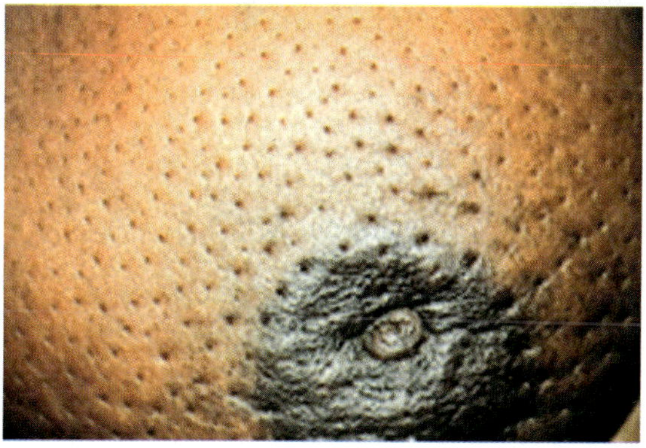

(a) Involvement of Cooper's ligament

(b) Blockage of subdermal lymphatics

(c) Involvement of connective tissue of breast

(d) Involvement of chest wall

*Image shows peau d'orange.*

*This is due to obstruction of dermal lymphatics; openings of the sebaceous glands and hair follicles get buried in the oedema giving rise to orange peel appearance.*

**Ans.: B i.e., Blockage of subdermal lymphatics**

*Reference: Page-569*

**18. A young male presented with severe abdominal pain and vomiting. He was sweating and have tachycardia. Per abdominal examination revealed a tender and rigid abdomen. Attending surgeon ordered a plain X-ray abdomen in erect posture, which is shown below. What is the best way to manage this patient?**

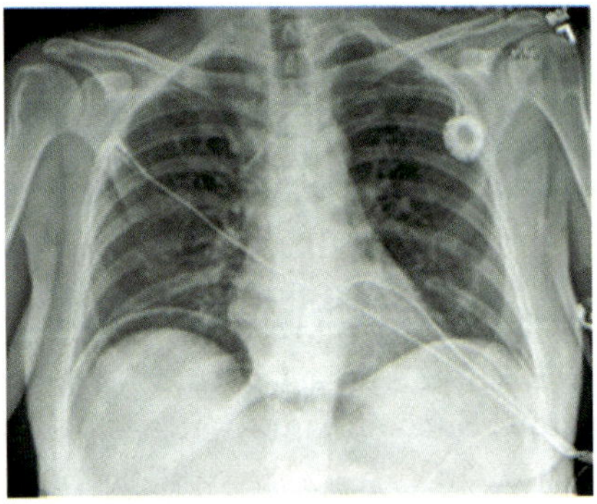

(a) Wait and watch

(b) I/V antibiotics

(c) Resuscitation and laparotomy

(d) USG whole abdomen

*Clinical presentation and X-ray are indicative of pneumoperitoneum (secondary to perforation).*

*Once perforation (peptic ulcer) occurs, contents of the gut escapes into the peritoneal cavity and cause chemical peritonitis leading to severe pain in the epigastric region, vomiting, tenderness, guarding, rigidity, tachycardia and sweating.*

*Plain X-ray abdomen (erect posture) shows gas under diaphragm in 70% of cases (can be seen on the right side in given X-ray).*

*Management include I/V fluids like Ringer lactate, antibiotics, catheterisation, Ryle's tube aspiration and emergency laparotomy through upper midline incision.*

**Ans.: C i.e., Resuscitation and laparotomy**

***Reference: Page-887, 888***

**19. Study the delayed intravenous urogram shown below and make a clinical diagnosis:**

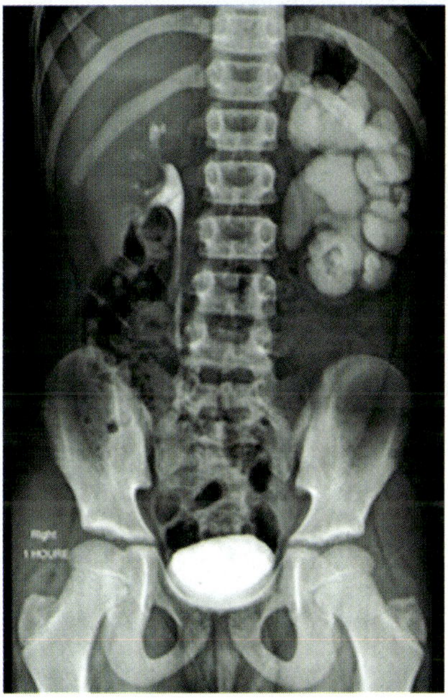

(a) Staghorn type of calculi

(b) Polycystic kidney disease

(c) Putty kidney

(d) Pelvi-ureteric junction obstruction

*Delayed IVU is indicative of hydronephrosis on left side.*

*One can see the clubbing of calyces.*

*Congenital PUJ obstruction is the most common cause of hydronephrosis.*

**Ans.: D i.e., Pelvi-ureteric junction obstruction**

***Reference: Page-1068, 1084***

**20. A young male had a road traffic accident and presented to the Emergency department with inability to pass urine. Vitals were stable. On examination, there was blood at the tip of urethral meatus. A retrograde urethrogram was done as shown below. Most likely site of urethral rupture:**

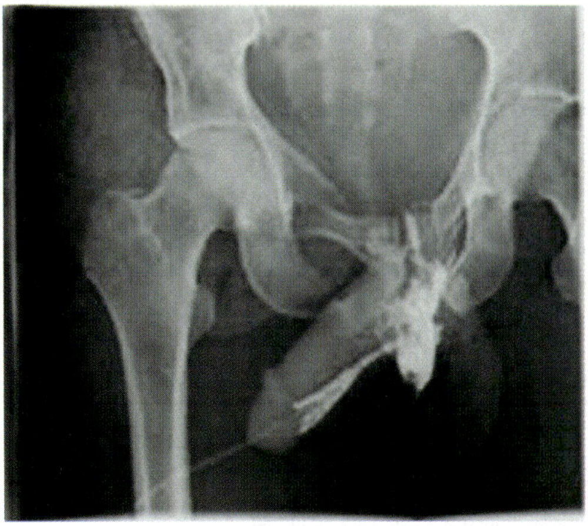

(a) Penile urethra (b) Bulbar urethra

(c) Membranous urethra (d) Prostatic urethra

*Clinical prestation and RGU are indicative of rupture of membranous urethra.*

*Posterior urethral rupture (membranous urethra and/or prostatic urethra) is usually associated with pelvic fracture (fractures of bilateral superior and inferior pubic rami can be seen in the image), commonly due to road traffic accidents.*

*Clinical features include blood in external meatus, failure of difficulty in passing urine and extravasation of urine to scrotum, perineum and abdominal wall.*

**Ans.: C i.e., Membranous urethra**

***Reference: Page-1129***

**21. A 50 years old female presented to the Surgery OPD with the complaints of single, smooth sweeling over the angle of mouth on left side. It was firm and painless. Clinical image is shown below. Most likely diagnosis:**

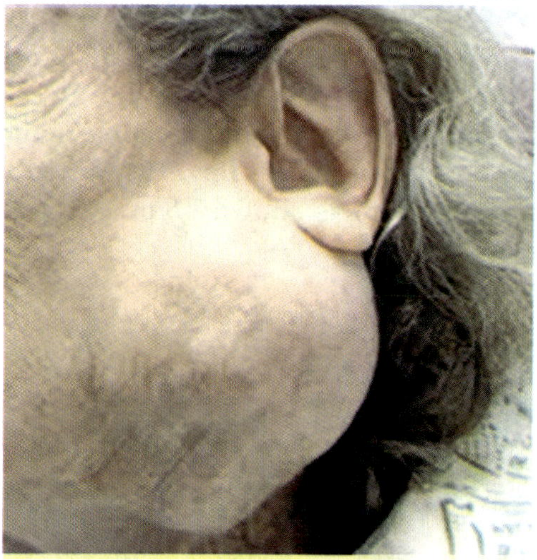

(a) Osteoma of the angle of mandible

(b) Parotid tumour

(c) Bezold's abscess

(d) Cervical lymphadenopathy

*Clinical presentation and image are indicative of parotid tumour.*

*Pleomorphic adenoma is the most common of the salivary gland tumour in adult.*

*Pleomorphic adenoma is common in females (3:1).*

*It can occur in any age but common in 4th and 5th decade.*

*Usually, unilateral.*

*Presents as a single painless, smooth, firm lobulated, mobile swelling in front of the parotid with positive curtain sign (As the deep fascia is attached above to the zygomatic bone, it acts as a curtain, not allowing the parotid swelling to move above that level. Any swelling superficial to the deep fascia will move above the zygomatic bone).*

*Obliteration of the retromandibular groove is common.*

*The ear lobule is lifted (seen in the given image).*

**Ans.: B i.e., Parotid tumour**

*Reference: Page-442*

**22. A road traffic accident patient with abdominal trauma was planned for emergency laparotomy. He was subjected to some investigation, as shown below. Identify the investigation:**

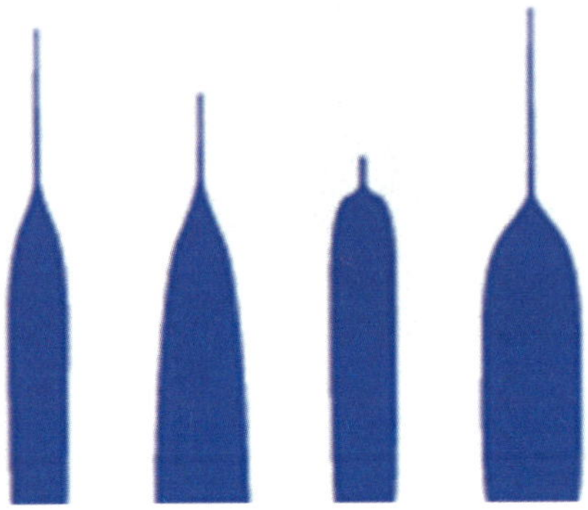

(a) Plethysmography (b) Thromboelastography

(c) Duplex scan (d) End tidal $CO_2$

*Thromboelastography (TEG) is a viscoelastic hemostatic assay that measures the global viscoelastic properties of whole blood clot formation under low shear stress.*

*TEG shows the interaction of platelets with the coagulation cascade (aggregation, clot strengthening, fibrin cross-linking and fibrinolysis).*

*It does not necessarily correlate with blood tests such as INR, APTT and platelet count (which are often poorer predictors of bleeding and thrombosis).*

**Ans.: B i.e., Thromboelastography**

***Reference: Internet resources***

**23. A young patient presented with jaundice. Laboratory test revealed a bilirubin of 21 mg/dl, conjugated bilirubin is 9.6 mg/dl and alkaline phosphatase is 450 IU/l. Most likely diagnosis:**

(a) Hemolytic jaundice

(b) Viral hepatitis

(c) Chronic active hepatitis

(d) Obstructive jaundice

*Markers in obstructive jaundice: Alkaline phosphatase is elevated (normal value is 20-140 IU/l), total serum bilirubin is elevated (normal value is 0.3-1 mg/dl) and conjugated serum bilirubin is also elevated (normal value is 0.1-0.4 mg/dl).*

**Ans.: D i.e., Obstructive jaundice**

*Reference: Page-697*

# OBSTETRICS

**1. While performing the procedure shown in the figure below, the umbilical cord got torn. What should be done next?**

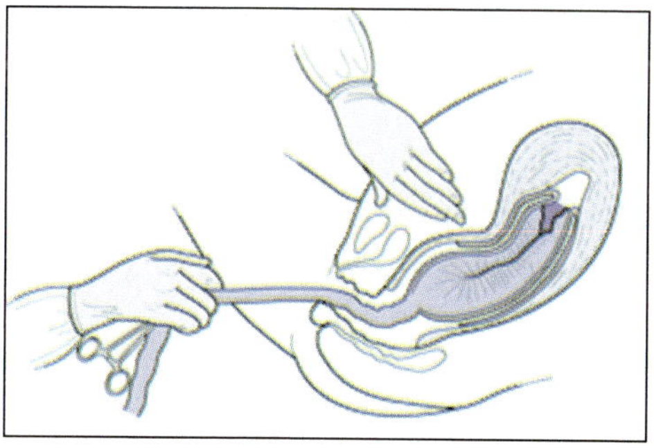

(a) Uterine massage

(b) Oxytocin drip

(c) Manual removal of placenta

(d) Arrange blood and deliver placenta by Crede's method

*Image shows controlled cord traction (modified Brandt-Andrews method) being done.*

*The cord may be accidentally torn which is not likely to cause any problem. The sterile gloved hand should be introduced, and the placenta is to be grasped and extracted.*

**Ans.: C i.e., Manual removal of placenta**

*Reference: Page-163*

**2. A primigravida pregnant lady was in labor with a fetus in right occipito-posterior presentation. Uterine contractions are good. Next step in management of such a patient:**

(a) Cesarean section

(b) Wait and watch for normal vaginal delivery

(c) Start oxytocin drip

(d) Forceps delivery

*In otherwise uncomplicated cases of occipito-posterior position, the labor is allowed to proceed in a manner similar to normal labor.*

*Favorable factor includes good uterine contractions and favorable pelvis (gynecoid).*

*Occipito-posterior position per se is not an indication of cesarean section.*

**Ans.: B i.e., Wait and watch for normal vaginal delivery**

*Reference: Page-430*

**3. The area drawn in green colour represents:**

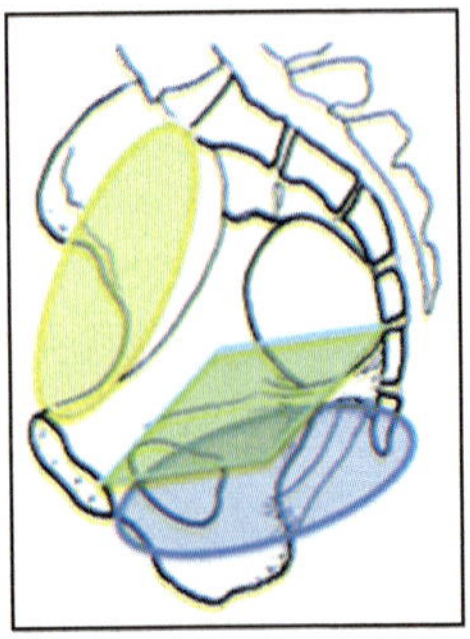

(a) Pelvic inlet (b) Obstetric outlet

(c) Anatomic outlet (d) Midpelvis

*Midpelvis is the segment of the pelvis bounded above by the plane of greatest pelvic dimensions and below by a plane known as midpelvic plane.*

**Ans.: D i.e., Midpelvis**

***Reference: Page-104***

**4. On 7th day of a normal vaginal delivery, a lady was brought to the emergency department at midnight with the complaints of loss of appetite, depression, difficulty in sleeping and occasional crying. General examination and pelvic examination were normal. What could be the most likely diagnosis?**

(a) Puerperal blues (b) Postpartum depression

(c) Postpartum psychosis (d) Postpartum insomnia

*Puerperal blues is observed 4-5 days after delivery and presents as depression, anxiety, tearfulness, insomnia, helplessness and negative feelings toward the infant.*

**Ans.: A i.e., Puerperal blues**

***Reference: Page-512***

**5. A 25 years old lady complains of right sided lower abdominal pain and mild bleeding per vaginum for one day after a period of amenorrhoea of 6 weeks. Her general condition is satisfactory and the vitals were stable. There is tenderness in the right iliac fossa. HCG level was 1400 IU/ml. Transvaginal ultrasound scan does not reveal any adnexal mass or any intrauterine pregnancy but the uterus was bulky and trilaminar endometrium was seen. There was no fluid in the pouch of Douglas. What is the next best step in management?**

(a) Perform a laparoscopic examination

(b) Repeat beta-HCG after 48 hours

(c) Repeat USG after a week

(d) Give progesterone

*Clinical history is indicative of an ectopic pregnancy since there is no intrauterine pregnancy.*

*A trilaminar appearance of endometrium has 94% specificity but 40% sensitivity to diagnose ectopic pregnancy.*

*Transvaginal sonography provides visualization of a well-formed intrauterine gestational sac as early as 4-5 weeks from the last menstrual period. The lowest level of serum beta-HCG at which a gestational sac is consistently visible using TVS (discriminatory zone) is 1,500 IU/l. The corresponding value of serum beta-HCG for transabdominal sonography is 6,000 IU/l.*

*(1) When the beta-HCG value is greater than 1,500 IU/l and there is an empty uterine cavity, ectopic pregnancy is more likely.*

*(2) Failure to double the value of beta-HCG by 48 hours along with an empty uterus is very much suggestive of ectopic pregnancy.*

*So, in the given MCQ, we would repeat the beta-HCG values after 48 hours to see whether it doubles or not. If it fails to double, then it's an indicator of ectopic pregnancy (as per criteria number 2).*

**Ans.: B i.e., Repeat beta-HCG after 48 hours**

*Reference: Page-213*

6. **A primigravida with full term pregnancy and in labor presented with sign and symptoms of dehydration. Her heart rate was 105 beats/minute, a BP of 130 /90 mm of Hg. Per abdominal examination showed a fundal height of 32 weeks, and the fetus was having right occipito transverse position. Fetal heart sounds were feeble and mild uterine contractions were felt. Per vaginal examination revealed a fully dilated cervix, head is at the level of ischial spine, caput was present and moulding was also present. Pelvis was found to be inadequate. What will be the most appropriate management of such a case?**

(a) Injection oxytocin

(b) Lower segment cesarean section

(c) Ventouse delivery

(d) Forceps application

*Clinical history suggests the diagnosis of deep transverse arrest.*

*The head is deep into the cavity; the sagittal suture is placed in the transverse bispinous diameter and there is no progress in descent of the head even after half to one hour following full dilatation of cervix.*

*When vaginal delivery is not found to be safe as in case of big baby or inadequate pelvis, perform cesarean section.*

*Operative vaginal delivery (Ventouse or forceps) for DTA should only be performed by a skilled obstetrician. Otherwise, cesarean delivery is always preferred.*

**Ans.: B i.e., Lower segment cesarean section**

*Reference: Page-431*

**7. A pregnant lady with 32 weeks pregnancy develops hypertension and edema. Urine examination shows presence of protein. Treating doctor suspected it to be a case of preeclampsia. Which of the following theory defines it:**

(a) Incomplete invasion of extra-villous cytotrophoblast into uterine artery

(b) Incomplete invasion of extra-villous cytotrophoblast into radial artery

(c) Incomplete invasion of extra-villous cytotrophoblast into basal artery

(d) Incomplete invasion of extra-villous cytotrophoblast into spiral artery

*Normally placenta has villi and intervillous spaces. The villi are lined by trophoblast and into the villi, open fetal blood capillaries.*

*In the intervillous space, spiral arterioles carrying maternal blood open.*

*The endovascular trophoblast replaces the lining of these maternal spiral arteries, making them low resistance, low pressure and high flow vessels.*

*In PIH, this trophoblastic invasion is incomplete, so maternal blood vessels have high resistance and high pressure causing PIH.*

**Ans.: D i.e., Incomplete invasion of extra-villous cytotrophoblast into spiral artery**

*Reference: Page-258*

8. **What will be the position of the uterus on 2nd postpartum day?**

   (a) At the level of umbilicus

   (b) Midway between umbilicus and pubis symphysis

   (c) Two fingers below umbilicus

   (d) Four fingers below umbilicus

   *There is no direct explanation to this MCQ. Let us try to derive our answer from the matter given in the textbook.*

   *Following delivery, the fundus lies about 13.5 cm (five and a half inch) above the pubis symphysis.*

   *During the first 24 hours, the level remains constant.*

   *Thereafter, there is a steady decrease in height by 1.25 cm (half an inch) in 24 hours.*

   *So, it means, on day 2 postpartum, uterus would remain more or less at the same height, which it attained at the time of labor (that is at the level of umbilicus). At the end of day 2, it would decrease in height by 1.25 cm (half an inch).*

   **Ans.: A i.e., At the level of umbilicus**

   ***Reference: Page-169, 170***

9. **A lady with pre-eclampsia presented to the Emergency department with absent patellar reflexes and bilateral plantar reflexes. She was having a respiratory rate of 11 breaths/minute and decreased urinary output. On auscultation, lung fields were clear. Her random blood sugar value was 210 mg/dl. Most likely diagnosis:**

   (a) Magnesium sulphate toxicity

   (b) Eclampsia

   (c) HELLP syndrome

   (d) Diabetes mellitus

   *Magnesium toxicity and serum magnesium levels: (a) Loss of deep tendon reflexes at more than 7 mEq/l; (b) Respiratory depression at more 10 mEq/l and (c) Cardiac arrest at magnesium levels of more than 25 mEq/l.*

**Ans.: A i.e., Magnesium sulphate toxicity**

*Reference: Page-273*

**10. A lady with 12 weeks of pregnancy presented for antenatal check-up. What would be your advice regarding calorie requirement?**

(a) 300 Kcal in second trimester

(b) 400 Kcal in second trimester

(c) 400 Kcal in third trimester

(d) 300 Kcal in all trimesters

*This is a very tricky question. Answer of this MCQ has to be made in relation to the patient given in this case. She had almost completed her first trimester, so obviously the word 'all trimesters' in this particular MCQ means second plus third trimester (first trimester cannot be taken into consideration while answering this particular MCQ).*

*The increased calorie requirement is to the extent of 300 over the non-pregnancy state during second half of pregnancy. The energy requirement in non-pregnant lady is 2200 Kcal, in pregnancy second half is 2500 Kcal and in lactating mother is 2600 Kcal.*

**Ans.: D i.e., 300 Kcal in all the trimesters**

*Reference: Page-112*

**11. A 26 years old primipara with normal BMI attended the antenatal clinic. She is having amenorrhoea of 35 weeks and a single live fetus in breech presentation. USG demonstrated complete breech presentation and adequate liquor volume. There was no other abnormality on USG scan. Her pregnancy is otherwise uncomplicated. What should be done next:**

(a) Perform an elective cesarean section at 39 weeks of pregnancy

(b) Perform an external cephalic version at 36 weeks of pregnancy

(c) Perform normal vaginal delivery at term

(d) Induction of labor, if not delivered till 40 weeks

*Everything is normal so ECV can be attempted. Successful version is likely in cases of complete breech, non-engaged breech, adequate liquor, sacroanterior posterior position (fetal back anteriorly) and non-obese patient.*

**Ans.: B i.e., Perform an external cephalic version at 36 weeks of pregnancy**

*Reference: Page-440*

**12. A 24 years old primigravida had postpartum hemorrhage, hypotension, shock and disseminated intravascular coagulation following normal vaginal delivery of a full-term healthy infant. Uterus is well contracted and hard. Fetus is normal. Most likely diagnosis:**

(a) Amniotic fluid embolism

(b) Ruptured uterus

(c) Vaginal laceration

(d) Uterine atony

*Features of shock and DIC goes in favour of the diagnosis of amniotic fluid embolism.*

*Liquor amnii is forced into the maternal circulation either through a rent in the membranes or placenta. Thromboplastin rich liquor amnii containing the debris, blocks the pulmonary arteries and triggers the complex coagulation mechanism leading to DIC.*

*Amniotic fluid embolism is one important cause of extracardiac shock in obstetrics.*

**Ans.: A i.e., Amniotic fluid embolism**

*Reference: Page-713, 703*

**13. A known case of cervical incompetence with previous abortion presented at 12 weeks of pregnancy. Doctor planned her for cerclage operation. Which of the following is an absolute contraindication for cervical cerclage operation?**

(a) Previous abortion

(b) Bag of water projecting into vagina

(c) Rupture of membranes

(d) Previous history of ectopic pregnancy

*Contraindications of cerclage operation: (i) Intrauterine infection. (ii) Ruptured membranes. (iii) Presence of vaginal bleeding. (iv) Severe uterine irritability. (v) Cervical dilatation greater than 4 cm. (vi) Fetal death or defect.*

**Ans.: C i.e., Rupture of membranes**

*Reference: Page-201*

**14. A 14 weeks pregnant lady was subjected to Color Doppler studies. By doing so, which of the following can be diagnosed?**

(a) Early onset pre-eclampsia

(b) Late onset pre-eclampsia

(c) Growth retardation

(d) Placenta accreta

*Doppler Ultrasound of high resistance index in the uterine artery (second trimester) is associated with sixfold increase in rate of preeclampsia. Presence of diastolic notch at 24 weeks gestation in the uterine artery can predict the possible development of preeclampsia.*

*Predictive factors for IUGR include abnormal uterine artery Doppler value (notching) at 20-24 weeks of pregnancy.*

*This seems a controversial question as the MCQ specifically mentions 14 weeks pregnancy and none of the conditions given in the options can be predicted/diagnosed so early, but since the word 'second trimester' is included in description for predicting preeclampsia, we can consider it as the answer.*

**Ans.: A i.e., Early onset pre-eclampsia**

*Reference: Page-264, 535*

**15. A lady with 22 weeks of pregnancy presented with lower abdominal pain and severe vaginal bleeding. A clinical diagnosis of unruptured ectopic pregnancy was made. Most likely site of implantation is:**

(a) Fallopian tube (b) Ovary

(c) Abdomen (d) Cervix

*Abdominal pregnancy can continue up to term.*

*Isthmic ectopic pregnancy rupture usually occurs at 6-8 weeks, the ampullary one at 8-12 weeks and the interstitial one at about 4 months.*

**Ans.: C i.e., Abdomen**

*Reference: Page-209*

**16. Which of the following is used for first trimester termination of pregnancy?**

(a) Intra-amniotic hypertonic urea

(b) Extra-amniotic saline infusion

(c) Oxytocin infusion

(d) Mifepristone and misoprostol

*Medical methods of first trimester MTP (up to 12 weeks) include: Mifepristone, Mifepristone and misoprostol, Methotrexate and misoprostol and Tamoxifen and misoprostol.*

*Surgical methods of first trimester MTP include menstrual regulation, vacuum aspiration, suction evacuation and/or curettage and dilatation and evacuation.*

**Ans.: D i.e., Mifepristone and misoprostol**

*Reference: Page-203*

**17. A 25 years old lady with a 24 months baby has heavy irregular bleeding during menstruation. The baby is on breast feed. Which of the following contraceptive agent is advised to such a patient?**

(a) Depot formulation (b) Cu-T 380A

(c) Progestasert (d) Mala-N

*Here we need to prescribe an agent, which serves 3 purposes: Contraception, relief in menorrhagia without affecting lactation.*

*Depot formulation/Injectable progestins include DMPA (like depot medroxy-progesterone acetate) and NET-EN (norethisterone enanthate).*

*Advantages: It can be used safely during lactation.*

*Menstrual symptoms, e.g., menorrhagia and dysmenorrhoea are reduced.*

**Ans.: A i.e., Depot formulation**

*Reference: Page-627*

**18. Blood test reports of a 24 weeks pregnant lady revealed AST and ALT >70 IU/l, bilirubin >1.2 mg/dl and platelet counts 90,000/mm$^3$. Most likely diagnosis:**

(a) Obstructive jaundice

(b) Viral hepatitis

(c) HELLP syndrome

(d) Dengue hemorrhagic fever

*HELLP syndrome is an acronym for Hemolysis, Elevated Liver enzymes and Low Platelets (below 100,000/mm$^3$). This is a rare complication of preeclampsia (10-15%).*

*Parenchymal necrosis of liver causes elevation in hepatic enzymes and bilirubin.*

**Ans.: C i.e., HELLP syndrome**

*Reference: Page-256, 258*

# GYNECOLOGY

**1. Which one of the following option is a contraindication for the use of contraceptive shown in the image?**

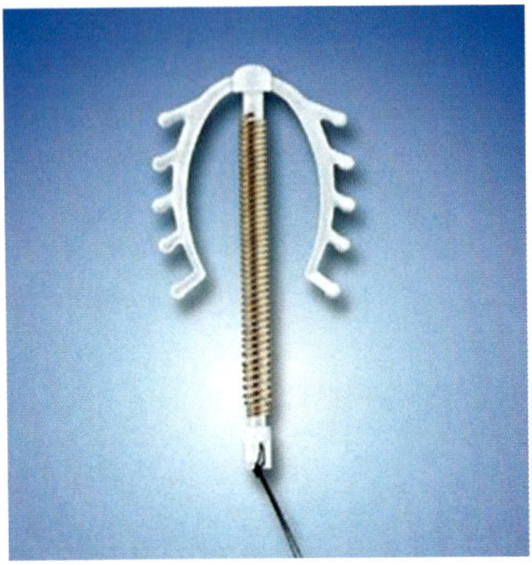

(a) Thromboembolic episode

(b) Undiagnosed genital tract bleeding

(c) Hypertension

(d) Breastfeeding women

*Image is of Multiload-375.*

*Contraindications for insertion of IUCD: (1) Presence of pelvic infection current or within 3 months; (2) Undiagnosed genital tract bleeding; (3) Suspected pregnancy; (4) Distortion of the shape of the uterine cavity as in fibroid or congenital uterine-malformation; (5) Severe dysmenorrhoea; (6) Past history of ectopic pregnancy; (7) Within 6 weeks following cesarean section; (8) Sexually transmitted illness – Current or within 3 months; (9) Trophoblastic disease; (10) Significant immunosuppression.*

**Ans.: B i.e., Undiagnosed genital tract bleeding**

***Reference: Page-480***

**2. A young lady was operated for Vesicovaginal fistula. As a doctor, what advice will you give her at the time of discharge?**

(a) Avoid intercourse for 1 month; Defer pregnancy for at least 6 months

(b) Avoid intercourse for 3 months; Defer pregnancy for at least 1 year

(c) Avoid intercourse for 6 months; Defer pregnancy for at least 2 years

(d) Avoid intercourse for 1 year; Defer pregnancy for at least 6 years

*Advice to be given to post-operative patient of VVF, during discharge: To pass urine more frequently, to avoid intercourse for at least 3 months, to defer pregnancy for at least 1 year and if conception occurs, to report to the hospital and must have mandatory antenatal check up and hospital delivery.*

**Ans.: B i.e., Avoid intercourse for 3 months; Defer pregnancy for at least 1 year**

*Reference: Page-423*

3. **Study the hysterosalpingogram given below and make a diagnosis:**

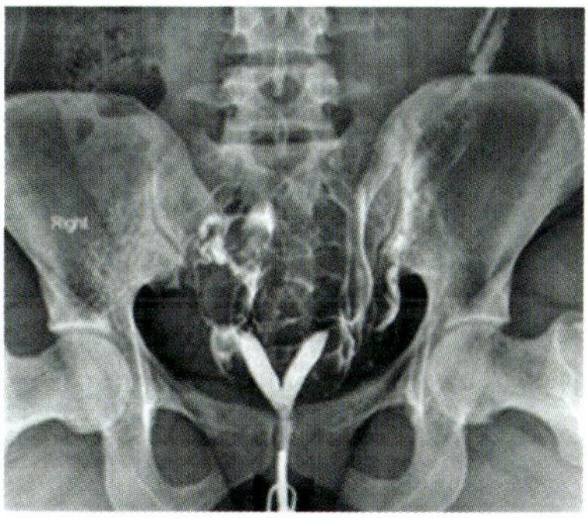

(a) Bicornuate uterus
(b) Septate uterus
(c) Uterus didelphis
(d) Uterus unicornis

*This seems a controversial question as it is difficult to differentiate between a septate and bicornuate anomalies on HSG, since the uterine fundal contour is not visible on HSG.*

*In the given MCQ, the two uterine cavities are widely separated so bicornuate uterus seems a better answer.*

**Ans.: A i.e., Bicornuate uterus**

*Reference: Page-45, 46, 658*

# DERMATOLOGY

1. **A known case of HIV is taking HAART. How to evaluate efficacy of treatment?**

   (a) Viral load

   (b) ELISA

   (c) p24 antigen

   (d) Western blot

   *HAART is an acronym for highly active anti-retroviral therapy (HAART).*

   *Accordingly, patients are treated with combination therapy of at least three antiretroviral drugs.*

   *This inhibits viral replication to below the limits of detection (< 50 RNA copies/ml).*

   *Viral load is now the preferred method of monitoring therapy. There should be more than or equal to 1 log reduction in viral load (reduction to less than 10,000 copies/ml, if pre-treatment viral load is 100,000 copies/ml) within 2-4 weeks after the commencement of treatment.*

   *If reduction in viral load is less than 0.5% log or stays above 100,000, then the treatment is adjusted by either adding or switching on to other drugs.*

   **Ans.: A i.e., Viral load**

   *Reference: Page-523*

2. **A patient presented with pitting of nails, subungual hyperkeratosis and oil drop changes. Clinical image is shown below. Most likely diagnosis:**

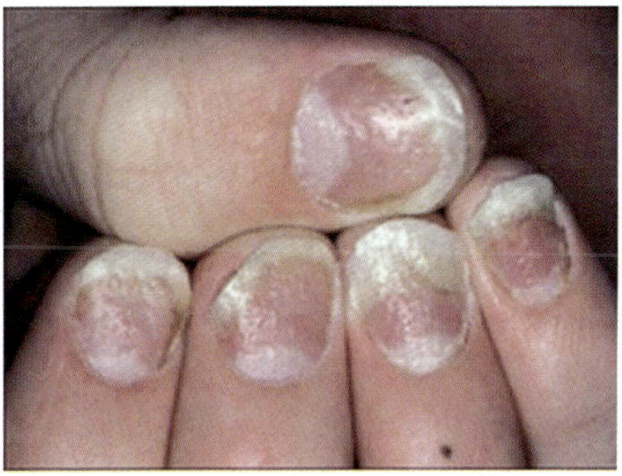

(a) Lichen planus (b) Psoriasis

(c) Onychomycosis (d) Tuberous sclerosis

*Clinical presentation and image are indicative of psoriatic nail changes.*

*Characteristically in psoriasis, there is coarse pitting of nails, discoloration and dystrophy of nail plate, subungual hyperkeratosis (accumulation of keratinous material under the nail plate), onycholysis (separation of distal part of the nail plate from nail bed), rounded areas of discoloration of nail bed may look like an oil drop, below the nail plate etc.*

**Ans.: B i.e., Psoriasis**

*Reference: Page-176*

**3. A known case of borderline tuberculoid leprosy was undergoing treatment. Which of the following nerve is commonly affected in such a case?**

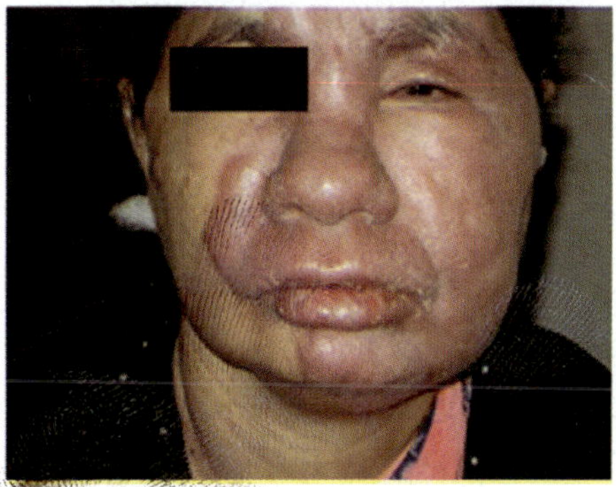

(a) 5th CN

(b) 7th CN

(c) Ventral rami of C2

(d) Transverse cervical nerve

*There is no direct explanation to this MCQ. Let us try to derive our answer from the matter given on the internet.*

*Among the cranial nerves, facial nerve was the most common nerve involved, followed by olfactory, trigeminal and auditory nerves.*

*Among the risk factors, it was found that facial nerve impairment was significantly associated with facial patch(es) and also type 1 lepra reaction.*

*Let us discuss few important features of borderline tuberculoid leprosy. The skin lesions are 2-3, which are well defined lesions. Satellite lesion is an important feature. Lesions are hypoesthetic and asymmetrical. Type 1 lepra reaction is seen.*

*Type 1 lepra reaction/delayed type hypersensitivity reaction/ reversal reaction is commonly seen in borderline (BT, BB) due to their unstable immunity.*

**Ans.: B i.e., 7th CN**

***Reference: Internet resources***

**4. A female presented to the Dermatology OPD with the complaints of hair loss for 3 weeks. She had a history of COVID-19 infection 3 months back. Most likely diagnosis:**

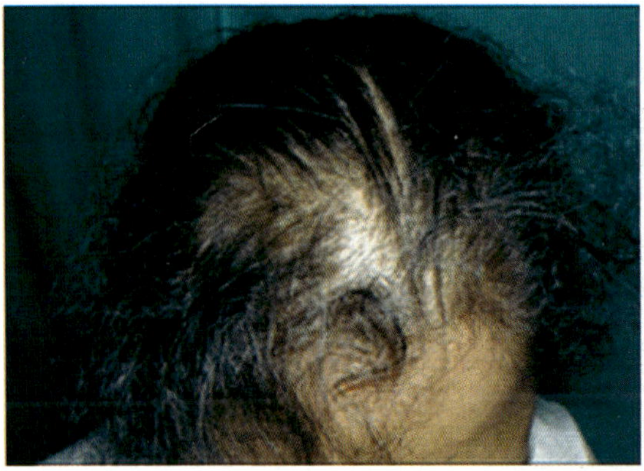

(a) Anagen effluvium (b) Telogen effluvium
(c) Trichotillomania (d) Alopecia areata

*Clinical presentation and image are indicative of Telogen effluvium.*

*Acute telogen effluvium is most common cause of diffuse hair loss in women followed by FPHL (female pattern hair loss) and chronic telogen effluvium.*

*The term "telogen effluvium" refers to excessive loss of club (telogen) hair in response to some unknown or known etiological factor.*

*This type of hair loss can be due to high grade prolonged fever (typhoid, dengue fever), child birth/abortion, major surgery, sudden starvation/crashing diet etc.*

*In telogen effluvium, 3-4 months after some inciting event, anagen phase terminates prematurely and there is a shift of fraction of anagen hairs to telogen.*

*Normally, anagen to telogen ratio is approximately 9:1 and 50 to 100 telogen hairs can be shed per day without causing alopecia.*

*In TE, this ratio shifts to 7:3 and 300 hairs are shed everyday.*

*Patient complaints of sudden, diffuse and excessive loss of scalp hair.*

**Ans.: B i.e., Telogen effluvium**

*Reference: Page-243*

5. **An obese lady presented to the Skin OPD with the complaints of dark patches over neck as shown in the figure. It is associated with:**

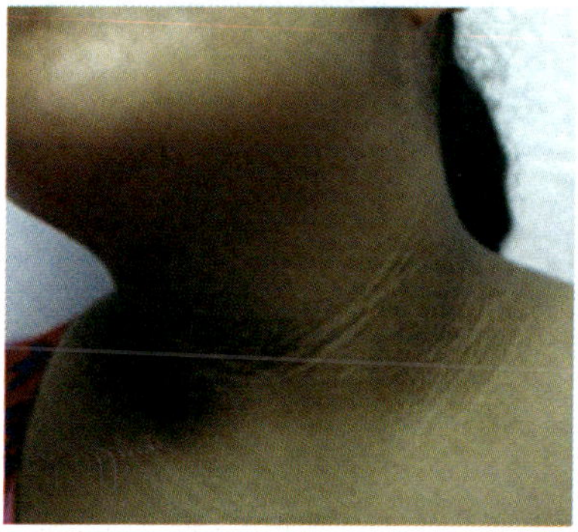

(a) Addison disease (b) Cushing syndrome

(c) Hypothyroidism (d) Metabolic syndrome

*Clinical presentation and image are indicative of acanthosis nigricans.*

*Acanthosis nigricans is characterised by typical velvety epidermal thickening with hyperpigmentation primarily in the axillary, inguinal and neck folds. Although severe AN can be associated with advanced malignant tumours, such as adenocarcinomas, it has been well associated with insulin resistance and diabetes mellitus.*

*Metabolic syndrome is not a disease in itself. Instead, it's a group of risk factors – high blood pressure (hypertension), high blood sugar (diabetes mellitus), unhealthy cholesterol levels and abdominal fat.*

**Ans.: D i.e., Metabolic syndrome**

***Reference: Page-346, Internet resources***

# ANESTHESIA

**1. Which nerve is tested to monitor neuromuscular blockade?**

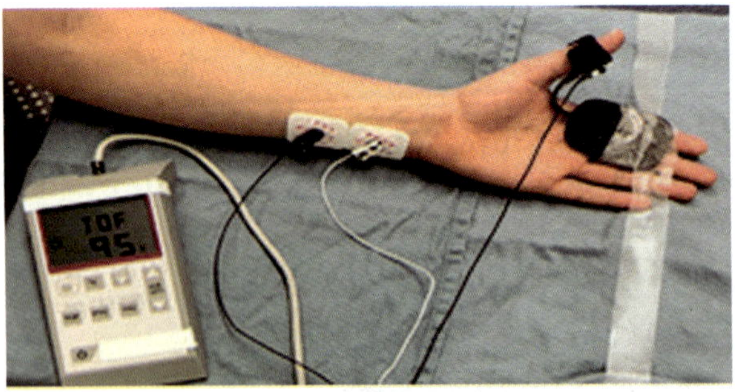


(a) Median nerve

(b) Ulnar nerve

(c) Radial nerve

(d) Posterior interosseous nerve

*Neuromuscular monitoring is required for patients suffering from neuromuscular diseases like myasthenia gravis, Duchenne's muscular dystrophy etc.*

*Most commonly used muscle for neuromuscular monitoring is adductor pollicis supplied by ulnar nerve.*

**Ans.: B i.e., Ulnar nerve**

***Reference: Page-54***

**2. Identify the equipment used commonly for COVID-19 patients:**

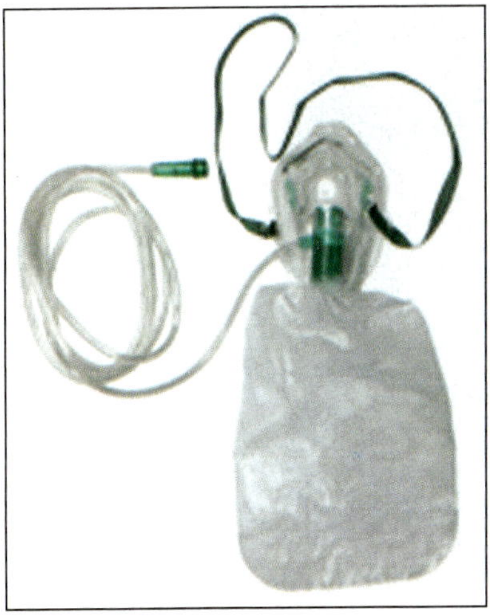

(a) Hudson mask

(b) Non-rebreather oxygen mask

(c) Venturi mask

(d) Laryngeal mask airway

*Non-breathing mask can deliver up to 80% of oxygen.*

**Ans.: B i.e., Non-rebreather oxygen mask**

***Reference: Page-43***

# RADIODIAGNOSIS & RADIOTHERAPY

1. **Identify the investigation shown below:**

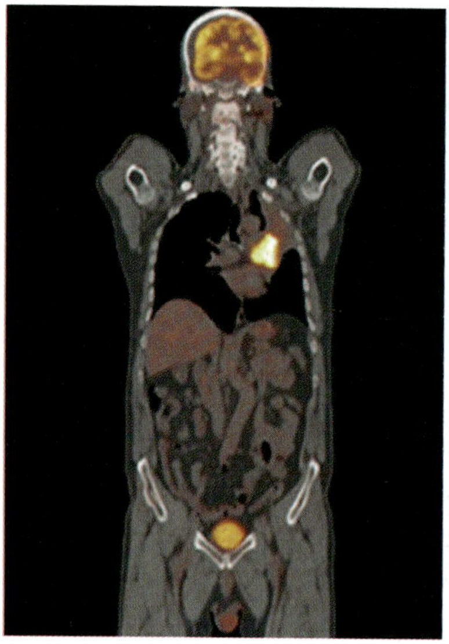

(a) Technetium scan (b) CT angiography
(c) PET-CT scan (d) DTPA

*PET-CT fusion scan has revolutionized onco-imaging, especially for follow-up of cancers.*

**Ans.: C i.e., PET-CT scan**

*Reference: Internet resources*

2. **A 30 years male smoker presented with pain in left foot and calf, which was of acute onset. His dorsalis pedis pulsations were feeble. Attending doctor advised for some investigation, which is shown below. Identify the radiological investigation:**

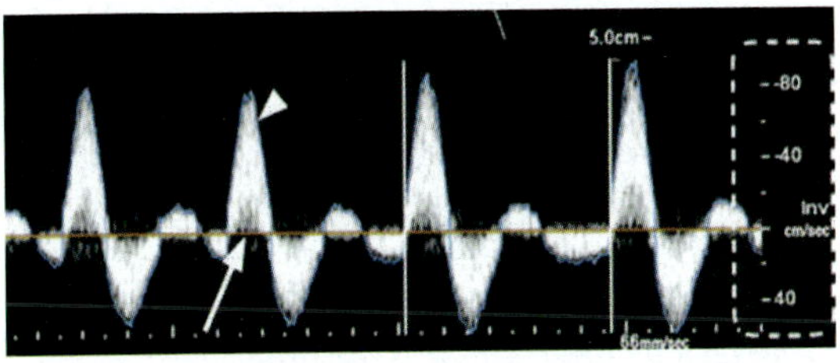


(a) Digital subtraction angiography

(b) MR angiography

(c) Ultrasound Doppler

(d) Plethysmography

*Clinical presentation is indicative of Buerger's disease and hence the patient was sent for colour Doppler study.*

*The Doppler effect is now commonly used in ultrasound imaging to examine the movement of liquids, such as blood flow in arteries and veins, allowing the location of blockage to be determined precisely.*

*When ultrasound is reflected from a moving surface, the frequency of the sound is altered slightly in a manner that depends on the speed of movement of the surface. This is due to the Doppler effect.*

**Ans.: C i.e., Ultrasound doppler**

*Reference: Page-33*

3. **A young patient presented with high grade fever, cough with purulent expectoration and difficulty in breathing. High Resolution CT of chest was done as shown below. Most likely diagnosis:**

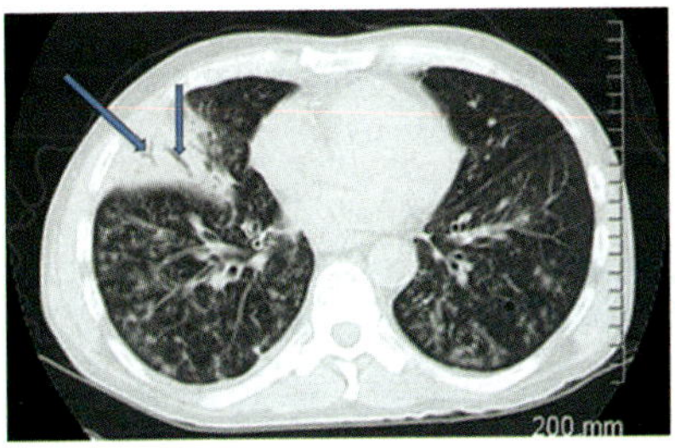


(a) Pleural effusion

(b) COPD

(c) Pulmonary sequestration

(d) Consolidation with air bronchogram

*Clinical presentation is indicative of pneumonia and HRCT is showing consolidation with air bronchogram.*

*Parenchymal lung consolidation may result in visualization of the intrapulmonary bronchi, which are otherwise not visible on normal chest radiograph. This occurs because the air within their lumens (blue arrows in the image) will then stand out in contrast to the surrounding opaque lung, know as air bronchogram.*

**Ans.: D i.e., Consolidation with air bronchogram**

*Reference: Page-97*

# PSYCHIATRY

**1. A 15 years old girl is having irresistible desire to eat. She also takes appetite suppressants. Most likely diagnosis:**

(a) Anorexia nervosa

(b) Bulimia nervosa

(c) Binge eating disorder

(d) Hysteria

*In bulimia nervosa, there is a persistent preoccupation with eating, and an irresistible craving for food. There are episodes of overeating in which large amounts of food are consumed within short periods of time (eating binges).*

*There are attempts to 'counteract' the effects of overeating by one or more of the following: self-induced vomiting, purgative abuse, periods of starvation, and/or use of drugs such as appetite suppressants.*

**Ans.: B i.e., Bulimia nervosa**

*Reference: Page-144*

**2. A patient was brought to the Emergency department by his relatives. He was having respiratory depression and**

**relatives suspected him to have overdosed with Opioids. Which drug is best used in managing such a case?**

(a) Naltrexone (b) Naloxone

(c) Flumazenil (d) Clonidine

*An overdose of opioid can be treated with narcotic antagonist (such as naloxone, naltrexone). Usually, an intravenous injection of 2 mg naloxone, followed by a repeated injection of in 5-10 minutes, can cause reversal of overdose. But as naloxone has a short half-life, repeated doses may be needed every 1-2 hours.*

*This seems a controversial question as both naloxone and naltrexone can be used for managing opioid overdose. But since description in the text is mainly for naloxone so we can consider naloxone as the answer.*

**Ans.: B i.e., Naloxone**

*Reference: Page-44*

# ORTHOPEDICS

1. **A child had a fall on ground over his left shoulder. After this he presented to the Emergency department with pain and swelling over left shoulder and he was supporting his left elbow with right hand. X-ray of the child is shown below. Which of the bone is fractured?**

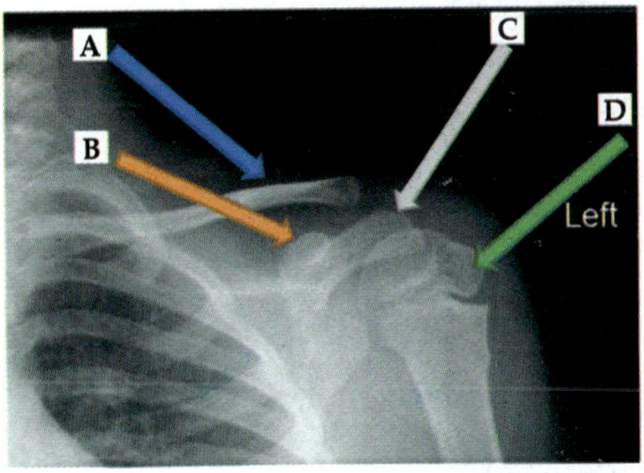

(a) A (b) B

(c) C (d) D

*X-ray shows an impacted fracture of proximal humerus (bone D). Fracture of the proximal humerus is usually caused by a fall on the shoulder. In majority of cases, these fractures are impacted.*

**Ans.: D i.e., D**

*Reference: Page-92*

2. **A $G_2P_1$ lady in the second trimester of pregnancy went for antenatal check-up. USG showed fractures in multiple long bones in the fetus. Fetus is suffering from:**

(a) Fetal hypothyroidism (b) Achondroplasia

(c) Osteogenesis imperfecta (d) Marfan syndrome

*Osteogenesis imperfecta is characterised by tendency for frequent fractures because of weak and brittle bones. It results from defective collagen synthesis.*

**Ans.: C i.e., Osteogenesis imperfecta**

*Reference: Page-317*

3. **A patient presented with multiple swellings in the right hand. X-ray suggest the diagnosis of:**

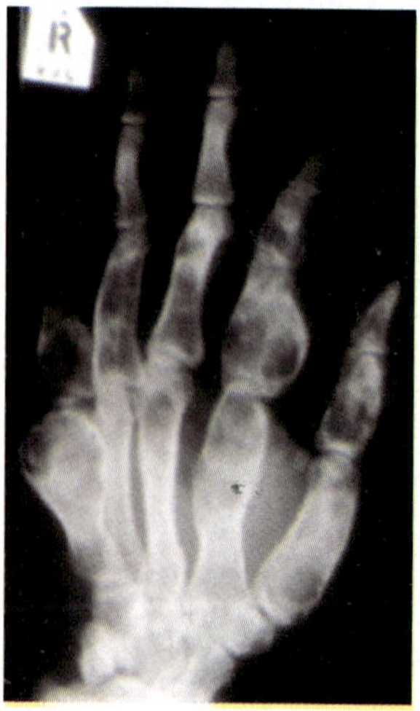

(a) Polyostotic fibrous dysplasia

(b) Multiple enchondromatosis

(c) Multiple brown tumours

(d) Multiple exostosis

*Enchondroma is a benign tumour consisting of lobulated mass of cartilage encapsulated by fibrous tissue. Small bones of the hands and feet are commonly affected. The presenting complaint is a long-standing swelling from one or more phalanges or metacarpals, without much pain.*

**Ans.: B i.e., Multiple enchondromatosis**

*Reference: Page-248*

4. **Identify the injury and the surgical procedure done as shown in the image below:**

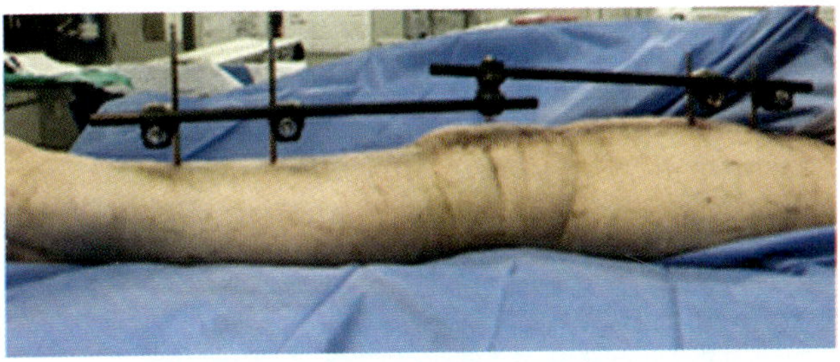

(a) Open fracture patella, Ilizarov fixator

(b) Fracture shaft tibia, Spanning fixator

(c) Fracture shaft femur, Spanning fixator

(d) Periarticular fracture of knee, Spanning fixator

*A joint-bridging/spanning external fixator is fixed to the femur and the tibia while the fracture zone is left virtually untouched (it is bridged). Provisional reduction is achieved with distraction.*

**Ans.: D i.e., Periarticular fracture of knee, Spanning fixator**

*Reference: Internet resources*

5. **What would be the best treatment plan for the injury in an adult, shown below in the X-ray?**

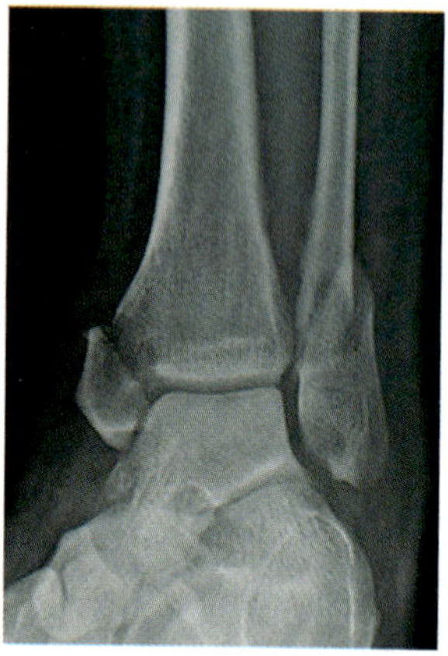

(a) Analgesic, Operative fixation

(b) Analgesic, Closed reduction, Cast

(c) Analgesic, Bed rest

(d) Analgesic, Neurological assessment

*X-ray shows displaced bimalleolar fracture. More and more surgeons are now resorting to internal fixation for all displaced fractures of ankle without attempting closed reduction. This is done because by operative reduction, it is possible to achieve perfect alignment as well as stable fixation of the fragments.*

**Ans.: A i.e., Analgesic, Operative fixation**

*Reference: Page-162*

**6. What could be the most common set of complications, if the injury shown in the X-ray below is not treated properly?**

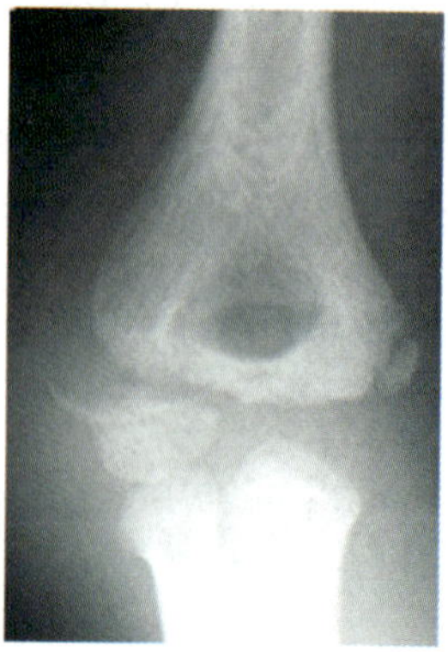

(a) Malunion, cubitus valgus deformity

(b) Malunion, cubitus varus deformity

(c) Non-union, cubitus varus deformity

(d) Non-union, cubitus valgus deformity

*X-ray shows displaced fracture of lateral humeral condyle. If unreduced, the fracture goes into non-union. This is either because of wide displacement of the fragments or a constant 'pulling' force of the extensor muscles attached to it. Diminished growth at the lateral side of the distal humerus epiphysis results in cubitus valgus deformity.*

**Ans.: D i.e., Non-union, cubitus valgus deformity**

***Reference: Page-103, 104***

7. **A child presented to the OPD with the complaints of pain in forearm and leg. X-ray showed diaphyseal sclerosis. Peripheral smear of the patient is shown below. Organism causing the bony problem in this child is:**

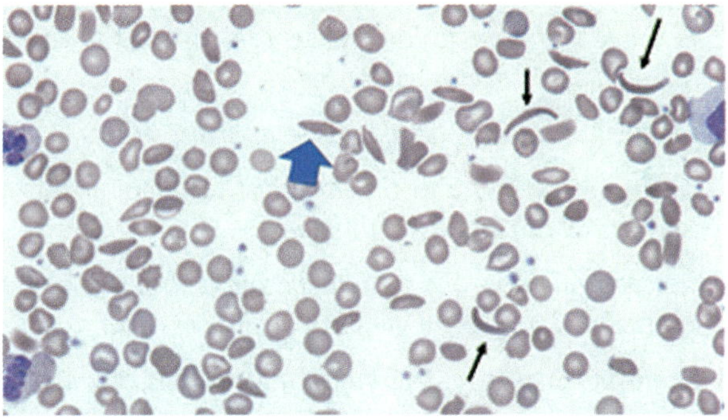

(a) Salmonella
(b) Staphylococcus
(c) Streptococcus
(d) E. coli

*Clinical presentation and image are indicative of salmonella osteomyelitis, which is seen in SCA patients.*

*This occurs during the convalescent phase after an attack of typhoid fever.*

*It is a subacute type of osteomyelitis, usually occurring in the ulna, tibia or vertebra.*

*Often, multiple bones are affected, sometimes bilaterally symmetrical.*

*The predominant radiological feature is a diaphyseal sclerosis.*

*The disease occurs more commonly in children with sickle cell anemia (sickle cell are shown by black arrows).*

**Ans.: A i.e., Salmonella**

*Reference: Page-175*

**8. A young male had a road traffic accident and presented to the Emergency with multiple injuries. After 2 days, he developed tachypnea, petechial rash and became drowsy. Most likely diagnosis:**

(a) Air embolism (b) Fat embolism

(c) Hemorrhagic shock (d) Pneumoperitoneum

*Clinical presentation is indicative of fat embolism.*

*FE is more common following severe injuries with multiple fractures and fractures of major bones.*

*Symptoms are evident in a day or so after the injury.*

*Presenting features are in the form of two, more or less distinct types: (1) cerebral; and (2) pulmonary.*

*In the cerebral type, the patient becomes drowsy, restless and disoriented and gradually goes into a state of coma.*

*In the pulmonary type, tachypnea and tachycardia are the more prominent features.*

*The other common features of fat embolism is a petechial rash, usually on the front of the neck, anterior axillary folds, chest or conjunctiva.*

**Ans.: B i.e., Fat embolism**

*Reference: Page-43*

# PEDIATRICS

1. **A 10 years old male child presented initially with peri-orbital edema and anasarca, later on. A clinical diagnosis of minimal change disease was made. Which of the following is true?**

   (a) Non-selective proteinuria

   (b) Commonly seen in adults

   (c) Steroid responsive

   (d) Light microscopy shows effacement of foot processes

   *Corticosteroids remain the mainstay of treatment of minimal change nephrotic syndrome for the initial episode as well as relapses.*

   **Ans.: C i.e., Steroid responsive**

   *Reference: Page-524 (Title 1)*

2. **On day 4, a neonate was found to have TSH >110 U/L. Ultrasonography revealed an eutopic thyroid gland. What should be done next?**

   (a) Thyroid nuclear scan

   (b) Anti-peroxide antibodies

   (c) Urinary iodine concentration

   (d) TSH receptors autoantibodies/TRab

   *Clinical presentation is indicative of congenital hypothyroidism.*

   *Estimation of thyroid hormones viz.* $T_4$*,* $T_3$ *and TSH is the mainstay for early diagnosis of congenital hypothyroidism.*

   *Both TSH and* $T_4$ *are raised on days 1 and 2 of life. So, the screening tests should be done between 3rd and 5th day of birth to decrease the false positive rates.*

   *USG examination of the thyroid is helpful for demonstration of thyroid tissue but it may fail to demonstrate some ectopic glands which may be shown by scintigraphy.*

*Scintigraphy with $^{123}$I-sodium iodide (thyroid nuclear scan) can help to pin point the underlying cause in infants with congenital hypothyroidism.*

*A normally situated thyroid gland with normal uptake radionuclide indicates a defect in the thyroid hormone biosynthesis.*

*Failure to demonstrate any thyroid tissue would suggest aplasia, TRab and iodine trapping defect.*

**Ans.: A i.e., Thyroid nuclear scan**

***Reference: Page-662, 663 (Title 1)***

3. **A mother was worried as her baby has not passed urine even after 20 hours of birth. What will be the next step?**

   (a) Start I/V fluids (b) Shift to NICU

   (c) Start formula milk (d) Wait and watch

   *The baby normally passes urine within 24-48 hours after birth.*

**Ans.: D i.e., Wait and watch**

***Reference: Page-167 (Title 1)***

4. **A 6 years old child presented with painful swelling of the hand and feet. There is a past history of chest infection 2 years back and he was admitted in the hospital too. Hemoglobin electrophoresis showed HbF and HbS. Most likely diagnosis:**

   (a) Beta-thalassemia

   (b) Anemic of chronic disease

   (c) Autoimmune hemolytic anemia

   (d) Sickle cell anemia

   *Clinical presentation is indicative of sickle cell anemia.*

   *Patient with SCA experience episodes which are traditionally called crises. There is vaso-occlusive crisis, sequestration crisis, aplastic crisis and hyperhemolytic crisis.*

   *The vaso-occlusive crisis presenting as 'hand foot syndrome' due to acute dactylitis is frequently the first overt evidence of sickle cell disease in an infant.*

*In SCA, HbS comprises 75-95% of total Hb, the rest being HbA (0%), $HbA_2$ (2-5%) and HbF (1-20%).*

**Ans.: D i.e., Sickle cell anemia**

*Reference: Page-281 (Title 1)*

5. **A 9 years old child presented to the Pediatrics OPD with the complaints of colicky abdominal pain and melena. On examination, palpable purpura was noted over buttocks and legs. Such a case should be treated by:**

(a) Cyclosporine (b) Corticosteroids

(c) Methotrexate (d) Cycloserine

*Clinical presentation is indicative of Henoch-Schönlein purpura.*

*It is characterised by purpuric rash, arthritis, abdominal pain and glomerulonephritis. The skin lesion is the most important sign.*

*Gastrointestinal symptoms occur in 75% of affected children. The most common complaint is colicky abdominal pain. In about 50% patients there is gross or occult blood in stool and hematemesis.*

*The skin lesions (purpura) usually appear on the lower extremities but may involve the buttocks, upper extremities, trunk and face as well.*

*There is no specific treatment for HSP. Systemic corticosteroids are indicated in patients with marked subcutaneous edema and severe rash, severe abdominal colic and orchitis.*

**Ans.: B i.e., Corticosteroids**

*Reference: Page-653, 654 (Title 1)*

6. **A child was subjected to routine hematological investigations and the peripheral blood smear showed microcytosis, hypochromia and target cells. His RBC indices were low MCV, low MCH. RBC count was $5.2 \times 10^9$/ microl. Which investigation should be done to arrive at a clinical diagnosis?**

(a) Serum homocysteine

(b) Serum ferritin

(c) $HbA_2$ estimation

(d) Red cell distribution width

*Clinical presentation is indicative of beta-thalassemia trait.*

*The condition is commonly not diagnosed until adolescence or adult life. It may be detected on routine hematological screening or when there is an affected child in the family with thalassemia major or a combination of HbE thalassemia or thalassemia S.*

*The hemoglobin level is normal or mildly reduced, rarely less than 10 gm%.*

*The peripheral blood smear shows mild red cell anisocytosis, microcytosis and hypochromia with variable number of target cells.*

*The RBC count is normal or increased despite anemia.*

*The MCV and MCH are reduced, with values of 63-77 fl and 18-25 pg respectively.*

*On electrophoresis, the most characteristic finding is an increase in $HbA_2$ (3.5-7%).*

**Ans.: C i.e., $HbA_2$ estimation**

***Reference: Page-288, 289 (Title 1)***

7. **A child born by normal vaginal delivery, had brief attacks of contraction of neck and trunk. There are jerky movements of hands as well. The episode is followed by crying. EEG showed hypsarrhythmia. Best drug to manage such a case:**

(a) Phenytoin (b) Phenobarbitone

(c) Carbamazepine (d) Injection ACTH

*Clinical presentation is indicative of infantile spasm.*

*Infantile spasm is a type of seizure characterized by brief symmetric contractions of neck, trunk and extremities.*

*A cry may precede or follow an infantile spasm.*

*The EEG most commonly shows hypsarrhythmia or a modified hypsarrhythmia pattern.*

*ACTH is the preferred drug for the treatment of infantile spasm.*

**Ans.: D i.e., Injection ACTH**

*Reference: Page-572 (Title 1)*

8. **A 3 years old child presented with anorexia, irritability and abdominal bloating. There is a history of passing foul-smelling stools which stick to the pan. The condition was associated with HLA DQ2. What is the best treatment for such a patient?**

(a) Low lactose in diet (b) Low gluten in diet

(c) High lactose in diet (d) High gluten in diet

*Clinical presentation is indicative of Celiac disease.*

*The disorder generally manifests a few months after the introduction of gluten containing food – often a wheat preparation in the feeding program.*

*Chronic diarrhoea – with large, pale, highly foul-smelling stools which stick to the pan (steatorrhoea).*

*Growth failure, anemia and other vitamin and nutritional deficiencies are seen.*

*Abdominal distension, irritability and anorexia are the usual presenting features.*

*HLA association include HLA-$DQ_2$ (DOA 1-*05/$DOB_1$/*$O_2$) or HLA $DO_8$ (DOA1*0301/DQBI*0302).*

*Besides symptomatic measures, the cornerstone of management is gluten withdrawal from the diet. Avoidance of wheat, barley, rye and oats in all forms brings about dramatic relief within weeks.*

**Ans.: B i.e., Low gluten in diet**

*Reference: Page-466 (Title 2)*

9. **An infant is having many episodes of vomiting and passing loose stools. He is lethargic and is not taking breastfeed. Skin when pinched goes back very slowly. Infant is having:**

(a) No dehydration (b) Mild dehydration

(c) Moderate dehydration (d) Severe dehydration

*Features of severe dehydration: Child is lethargic/unconscious, eyes are very sunken and dry, tears are absent, mouth and tongue are very dry, patient is not able to drink and on skin pinch, skin goes back very slowly (takes more than 2 seconds).*

**Ans.: D i.e., Severe dehydration**

***Reference: Page-372t (Title 1)***